A Historical Introduction to Mathematical Modeling of Infectious Diseases

A Historical Introduction to Mathematical Modeling of Infectious Diseases

Seminal Papers in Epidemiology

Ivo M. Foppa

Adjunct Associate Professor, Emory University, Atlanta, GA, United States

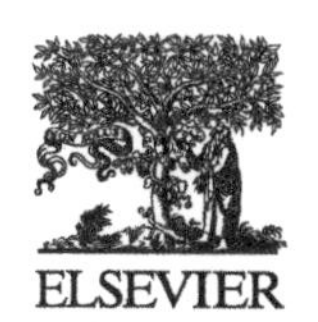

AMSTERDAM • BOSTON • HEIDELBERG • LONDON • NEW YORK
OXFORD • PARIS • SAN DIEGO • SAN FRANCISCO • SINGAPORE
SYDNEY • TOKYO
Academic Press is an imprint of Elsevier

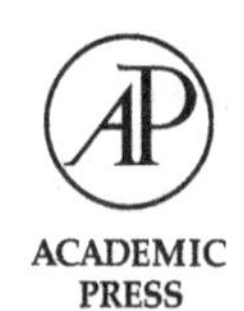

Introduction

Motivation and short history (of this book)

In general, the motivation for a book, as well as its history, is "meta-information". At least in fictional literature, such aspects of a book may be revealed and evaluated by critics, but for the reader it should have little relevance. This may, in general, be particularly true for textbooks. There, the substance of the material presented and manner in which it is presented are of sole relevance except, perhaps, for its cost.

In the case of the book that you are, at least figuratively, holding in your hands, I beg to disagree: I believe that for this book the *motivation* behind it certainly matters. To put the motivation into context, I have to reveal some autobiographical history.

In 1994, I enrolled at the Harvard School of Public Health in Boston, MA, in a one-year Master of Science program in *Epidemiologic Methods*. I had specifically chosen that program, as I had muddled through as a research epidemiologist for a few years, constantly and sorely aware of my lack of a solid epidemiological background. I desperately wanted to understand what I was doing and was lucky enough win a Scholarship of the Swiss National Science Foundation. At the time, there were no opportunities to study epidemiology in Switzerland, or any other field of public health. The need to train a public health work force was clearly perceived and the mentioned funding mechanism was chosen as a temporary solution to the problem.

During the Spring semester of my first year, the third term of that academic year to be exact, I enrolled in a course with the, quite unassuming, title "Epidemiology of Infectious Diseases." It was taught by Dr. Jonathan Freeman, a physician with a doctorate in epidemiology from the same department he was now a faculty member of. He used graphs of numerical solutions to simple ordinary differential equation models to illustrate the key features of infectious disease transmission (Fig. 1). He was, by no means, an "infectious disease modeler", but he had been acquainted with this method relatively recently himself and was full of enthusiasm for the intriguing possibilities. To me, this was truly eye-opening, and I discovered my deep fascination with infectious disease transmission dynamics. During the following term, Freeman taught a follow-up course that was entitled something like "Epidemiologic Analysis of Outbreaks of Infectious Diseases" which focused less on transmission modeling as a tool, but taught more specific epidemiologic characteristics of important types of infectious diseases. In that course, I also met Andrew Spielman, Professor at the Department of Immunology and Infectious Diseases (then "Department of Tropical Public Health") an important and visionary public health entomologist who gave a lecture on the emergence of Lyme disease in the Atlantic Northeast. Spielman, by the way, had identified the tick *Ixodes dammini* as the vector of Lyme disease in the Northeast [4]; today, the identity of *Ix. dammini* is no longer widely recognized, but rather lumped together with the tick *Ix. scapularis*, a behaviorally quite different tick.

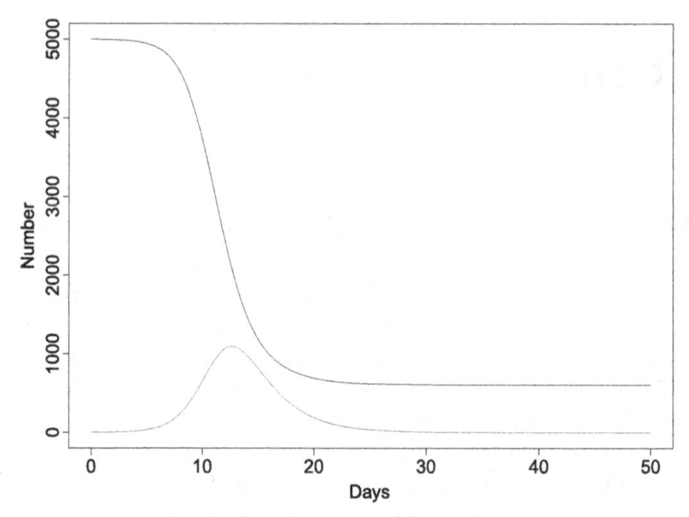

Figure 1 Outcome of a "synthetic" epidemic: Numerical solution of a simple susceptible–infectious–removed (= SIR) epidemic (see, for example, Chap. 4) in a closed population. The top line (blue in the online version of the Figure) represents the number of susceptibles and the bottom line (red in the online version of the Figure) the number of infecteds over time. Even though this "outbreak" relies on some simplifying and even unrealistic assumptions, the shape of the epidemic curve (bottom, red in online version) closely resembles data from real disease outbreaks.

Spielman would argue that the denial of the species identity of *Ix. dammini* was due to a scientific blunder.

Be it as it may, this educational experience encouraged me, after I had been admitted to the doctoral program, to pursue research in infectious diseases, tick-borne disease transmission dynamics, to be precise. Jonathan Freeman became my doctoral advisor, Andrew Spielman the second reader of my dissertation.

Freeman's class incited my keen interest in problems of infectious disease transmission dynamics. This would remain the only formal education I received in that area and the training was mostly conceptional, providing little exposure to mathematical and technical aspects of mathematical modeling. I therefore acquired most of that material myself. I first read Roy Anderson and Robert May's "Infectious Diseases of Humans: Dynamics and Control" [1], a very influential book that profoundly shaped the perception of models of infectious disease transmission by "popularizing" the topic. Anderson and May achieved that *popularizing* effect through their very readable presentation of the most important results in the field and their interpretation as to the implications of these results for public health practice. Freeman encouraged his students to read that book—it was, in fact, required reading for his "Epidemiology of Infectious Diseases" class.

Reading *the* Anderson and May motivated me to take a look at some of the important sources they discussed. In fact, I had begun to develop a certain level of distrust of secondary sources, a sentiment that increasingly led me to the *original* sources. Kermack and McKendrick's groundbreaking 1927 paper [3] (see Chap. 4) was one of the first targets of my quest. I was dismayed at the high level of mathematical expertise that seemed necessary to fully understand that paper; I certainly was not mathematically prepared. I also noted how little the paper seemed to be reflected in Anderson and May's interpretation of it.

My odyssey through the "classical papers" that was driven by my desire to more fully understand often met obstinate obstacles. Repeatedly, weeks went by when I remained stranded at single lines of mathematical expressions, without the slightest clue as to how they were derived and what they meant. Ultimately, however, I reached the point of understanding every time, sometimes after frustrating and often tortuous searches for the necessary pieces of knowledge. Each time, the satisfaction of successfully deciphering the "code" was reward enough to continue.

During my, often painfully slow, journey I was forced to realize that my modest mathematical background did not prepare me well for my endeavor. Unfortunately, some of the authors did not offer any proverbial hand to the reader, to help him or her navigate those "treacherous passages". Instead, they unnecessarily—sometimes there almost seemed to be mischievous intent—obscured the trail, leaving readers like myself struggling desperately. Whether the occasional preface to these passages, such as "it is easy to see" or "it can easily be shown" merely reflected their mischief or even some confusion on their part is beyond my knowledge. Occasionally, I discovered inconsistencies if not mistakes in some of those famed writings. These were never appreciated in the secondary literature.

After years of this pursuit an idea started to germinate: Maybe I could try to convey what I had learned and offer that hand when the authors did not. This would make my own struggles worthwhile. Thus the idea to this book was born.

Structure and suggested use of the book

All of the seven chapters of this book are devoted to one (Chaps. 1, 2, 4), two (Chaps. 3, 5, 7) or four (Chap. 6) papers or passages from books.

The chapters are presented in rough chronological order. That order is not always precise as some of the companion articles, for example, the ones from Chaps. 3 or 5 are temporally separated by decades. What joins the papers within a chapter, however, is their topic or even approach.

Ideally, the reader should have access to copies of the discussed papers. Unfortunately, I cannot grant this access, due to copyright restrictions. However, most university libraries should be able to provide access. In addition, many of the resources can be obtained free of charge on the Internet. Reading these papers while following the text of the book would be optimal, even though this is not absolutely necessary. In most cases, however, I work through only parts of papers; the perusal of their remainders certainly may be of interest to the readers.

The text of the chapters is organized as follows:

- A short introduction sets the stage for the mathematical derivations. Very little historical context or background is provided beyond what is absolutely essential. The book by Bacaër [2] examines some of the same papers discussed here, taking a very different approach; much more context information is provided there.

- The main mathematical arguments are followed and derived, using a measured step-by-step tour through derivations and expressions. The procedures are explained in great detail in the text, and the mathematical equations are commented on as illustrated by an example from Chap. 6:

$$\begin{aligned}
n &= \frac{n+1}{1+(n+1)C} \text{ (time } t=0\text{, so the exp falls away)},\\
1+(n+1)C &= \frac{n+1}{n} \text{ (multiply by right denominator and divide by } n),\\
(n+1)C &= \frac{n+1}{n} - 1 \text{ (subtract 1 from both sides)},\\
(n+1)C &= \frac{1}{n} \text{ (note that } \frac{n+1}{n} - 1 = \frac{n+1}{n} - \frac{n}{n} = \frac{n+1-n}{n}),\\
C &= \frac{1}{n(n+1)} \text{ (divide both sides by } (n+1)).
\end{aligned}$$

The development of the mathematical argument forms the "backbone" of the text.

- The text is inter-dispersed with questions. Here is an example from Chap. 5:

Question 5.h

Derive the corrected equilibrium value of x according to model (5.22).

Answers are proposed at the end of each chapter. Often, there is no single best answer. Here is the answer to the example question above:

Answer 5.h

If we set Eq. (5.22) to zero, calling the equilibrium value of x as L, we get

$$\begin{aligned}
0 &= h(1-L) - rL,\\
h(1-L) &= rL,\\
h - hL &= rL,\\
h &= rL + hL \text{ (adding } hL \text{ to both sides)},\\
h &= L(r+h) \text{ (factoring } L),\\
\frac{h}{r+h} &= L.
\end{aligned}$$

Therefore,

$$L = \frac{h}{r+h}.$$

These questions are thought to stimulate the independent and critical thinking of the reader and to help solidify the insights gained.

- Beyond guiding the reader through the mathematical arguments, very few explanations are given regarding the *interpretation* of mathematical insights in the context of the larger public health problem studied. This is, after all, not something this book pretends to convey.

Target audience

This book is not a textbook in the usual sense, but has been conceived to be an empowering tool for readers who are not sufficiently prepared to immediately understand the key papers on the foundation of which modern transmission modeling is based. The empowering message I intended to convey is as follows: A deep understanding and critical appreciation of these "classical" texts can be achieved despite their sometimes obscure presentation and despite a reader's modest mathematical foundation. Mathematics may be the queen of sciences, but she should never be used to obscure the goals she is supposed to help reach.

The intended audience for this book is anybody striving to learn mathematical modeling from basic principles, who has the patience and tenacity to persist through the tedium, and especially who had little mathematical formation beyond the high school level. Readers with a strong mathematical background may be less dependent on the step-wise and often tedious instructions that are intended to help the less equipped. They may even be bored by that aspect or criticize a certain lack in mathematical rigor. Even those readers, however, may profit from the in-depth analysis to develop an understanding of the meaning of the mathematical results for specific problem studied.

Graduate students of epidemiology or related subjects may be able to take advantage of this book, as might be self-directed students of mathematical epidemiology. From teaching epidemiology at the graduate level for years, I derive a high level of confidence that many, if not most, epidemiologists striving to understand the classical papers dealing with modeling infectious diseases will struggle, just as I did.

I encourage and try to foster a critical appreciation of the work being analyzed that does never assume infallibility in the texts studied.

Mathematical background

Ideally, readers should have a solid high school level mathematics background. Basic knowledge of calculus is needed to follow much of the arguments. For readers having never had an opportunity to study calculus, numerous online and offline resources could be used to acquire very basic knowledge of calculus. An essential truth: Everything can be learned with some effort. For most readers, the effort required to fully follow this book should be modest. Nevertheless, a certain enjoyment of mathematical concepts and appreciation of mathematical reasoning is paramount.

Miscellaneous remarks

1. The approach of this textbook is novel and thus unique; whether it works and provides access to not very accessible material or whether it is too tedious to be of any true benefit remains to be seen.
2. Some of the papers discussed here are of undoubted prominence, such as the one by Kermack and McKendrick [3] or the paper by van den Driessche and Watmough [5]. Nevertheless, the selection of articles was necessarily, to some extent, arbitrary.
3. Several topics that I would have liked to discuss could not be fit into the book for reasons of time (to complete the work) and space (in terms of pages). The most important among these topics is the statistical analysis of data from infectious disease outbreaks. This topic was neglected for a long time, but due to developments—both in computational power and statistical theory—exciting methods emerged over the past two or so decades. There is a strong connection with, in particular stochastic, transmission models.
4. I have tried to avoid mathematical errors, but the arguments I develop as well as the explanations I give lack formal rigor. Yet, they should serve their intended purpose well, empowering the reader to understand.

References

[1] R.M. Anderson, R.M. May, B. Anderson, Infectious Diseases of Humans: Dynamics and Control, vol. 28, Wiley Online Library, 1992.
[2] N. Bacaër, A Short History of Mathematical Population Dynamics, Springer Science & Business Media, 2011.
[3] M. Kermack, A. McKendrick, Contributions to the mathematical theory of epidemics. Part I, Proceedings of the Royal Society. Series A, Containing Papers of a Mathematical and Physical Character 115 (1927) 700–721.
[4] A. Spielman, C.M. Clifford, J. Piesman, M.D. Corwin, Human babesiosis on Nantucket Island, USA: description of the vector, Ixodes (Ixodes) dammini, n. sp. (Acarina: Ixodidae), Journal of Medical Entomology 15 (3) (1979) 218–234.
[5] P. Van den Driessche, J. Watmough, Reproduction numbers and sub-threshold endemic equilibria for compartmental models of disease transmission, Mathematical Biosciences 180 (1) (2002) 29–48.

Acknowledgments

I would like to acknowledge a few people: My colleague and friend Manoj Gambhir, Associate Professor, Head of the Epidemiological Modelling Unit, Department of Epidemiology and Preventive Medicine, Monash University, Melbourne, Australia, graciously gave me a few very useful hints, especially when I was stuck in some of Kermack and McKendrick's mathematical arguments. Rhys Griffiths, Acquisition Editor at Elsevier helped me get the book project off the ground. His professional behavior and approachable demeanor starkly contrasted with my experience with another major publisher, whose acquisition editor simply left me hanging. When Rhys left Elsevier, I was "adopted" by Molly McLaughlin, Editorial Project Manager at the Massachusetts Office and Erin Hill-Parks, Acquisition Editor at the London Office. Both Molly and Erin showed seemingly endless patience towards me and were always extremely responsive to my many requests and inquiries and were instrumental to bringing this project to an end. I would also like to thank the Senior Project Managers, Karen East and Kirsty Halterman being so helpful fixing technical problems in the final phase and everybody else in the background helping to realize this book. Last but not least I would like to express my gratitude towards all people, such as Paul Dawkins of Lamar University ("Paul's Online Math Notes", http://tutorial.math.lamar.edu/), but also "institutions", such as Wikipedia or MITOPENCOURSEWARE (http://ocw.mit.edu/index.htm) for making a treasure trove of mathematical knowledge available to the public—without them, I would not have succeeded.

Acknowledgment

D. Bernoulli: A pioneer of epidemiologic modeling (1760)

1

Contents

1.1 Bernoulli and the "speckled monster"

Smallpox likely emerged in prehistoric times. By the end of the Middle Ages, the disease became a constant presence in population centers of Europe and Asia, causing substantial child mortality. The term "speckled monster" bears witness to the life-threatening presence of the disease. Even though its etiology was not elucidated until the early 20th century, it became the first infectious disease against which a specific intervention was available, variolation or inoculation. This intervention consisted of the administration of pustulous material from a smallpox patient to a "healthy" person, typically a child. A typically mild form of smallpox infection ensued that conferred livelong immunity to the disease. Bernoulli eloquently sets the stage for his question: How would the world look like if everybody were inoculated?

The following analysis is largely based on the original text of Bernoulli's Mémoire [1]. Bradley [3] published a commented English translation, referring to the paper as a

> *"[. . .] first attempt at a mathematical theory of the propagation of an infectious disease".*

As we will see, this assessment is not quite accurate. Except for a few passages, the translation is excellent and helpful to English speakers with insufficient knowledge of French. Bernoulli's article is also accessible in English in the reprint presented by Blower [2]. Insightful comments on Bernoulli's contribution were also published by Dietz and Heesterbeek [4,5].

The main text of the *Mémoire* is structured into 21 paragraphs (§1–§21) and cumulates in two tables, presented at the very end. In the "vindicatory introduction"

A Historical Introduction to Mathematical Modeling of Infectious Diseases. DOI: 10.1016/B978-0-12-802260-3.00001-8 which was written about five years after the Mémoires, Bernoulli responds to some of his critics, and it is interesting to read. However, I will focus on the main text here.

1.1.1 §1 through §4: Preamble

Bernoulli comments on the assumed fraction of the total mortality of each generation that is attributable to smallpox and states that he has seen mortality lists indicating $\frac{1}{14}$ and others supporting $\frac{1}{13}$. It is not quite clear how he used these lists to calculate these fractions. It becomes evident in §2 that he counted the smallpox deaths over an indeterminate succession of years and divided that by the total number of deaths.

Question 1.a

Consider the ratio, $\frac{d_s}{d_T}$, where d_s represents the deaths due to smallpox, and d_T are the total deaths. Does that ratio represent the proportion dying of smallpox in each generation?

Most of the remainder of that paragraph (§1) is devoted to a peculiar justification of inoculation. Bernoulli states that, by observing case fatality rates as low as $\frac{1}{40}$, it seems quite natural to him to presume that the fatality of smallpox depends less on the state of its victims than on the "more or less malign character of the cause which produces it".[1] He thus justifies the harmlessness of inoculation when administered in inter-epidemic periods. While this reason, from today's perspective, appears quite abstruse, we have to consider the fact that the "germ theory" of infection was not proven until a century later and the smallpox virus was characterized only in the early 20th century. This did not prevent Bernoulli from getting the epidemiologically important aspects of the disease right, namely that it was an infectious phenomenon and that infection resulted in life-long immunity. A quite important aside: The clinical manifestation of smallpox was so unique that the label of "smallpox" was, despite the absence of modern diagnostic criteria, generally quite accurate.

The second paragraph (§2) is mostly devoted to the question of the overall proportionate mortality ratio of smallpox and variations thereof. Most contemporary estimates ranged from $\frac{1}{14}$ (England) to $\frac{1}{10.5}$ (Breslaw). Bernoulli attributes the variability in these estimates and our insufficient knowledge of this proportion to numerical reasons:

> *"If we knew exactly the mean proportions as calculated from a very great number of observations [...] we could develop a complete theory of the hazards of smallpox. Such a theory would dictate the rules all reasonable people would have to follow."*

[1] In the original: "*[...] la nature plus ou moins maligne de la cause qui la produit [...].*"

Question 1.b

According to his quote, Bernoulli speculated that the elusiveness of the "hazards of smallpox", i.e. the risk of acquiring it and of dying from it, were only due to the limitations of contemporary observations. This statement appears to suggest that observations in "very high" numbers would lead to stable estimates of these hazards (to die from smallpox). Does this reflect a modern view of the epidemiological process?

Bernoulli, in §3, then introduces two parameters that, at the time, were poorly characterized[2]:

- The annual risk of acquiring smallpox at each year of life;
- The case fatality ratio.

The exact knowledge of these two parameters, that Bernoulli deems more easily obtained for the second one, would, as he states, allow him to accurately construct a counterfactual world without smallpox. The first subparagraph, which is devoted to the first parameter, conveys Bernoulli's great and important insight. He will, for the remainder of the *Mémoire*, assume that, independently of age, in n persons not yet touched by smallpox, one person will acquire it on average in the course of a year. Bernoulli writes that

> *"according to this hypothesis, the hazard of acquiring smallpox remains the same for each year of life as long as one has not yet acquired it."*

Let, for example, $n = 10$. The annual risk of any person to suffer from smallpox therefore will be $\frac{1}{10}$ until he or she has acquired it. Bernoulli then states, somewhat ambiguously, that the probability of a person to have suffered smallpox after a given year decreases until a person has acquired it.[3] This latter passage is mistranslated by Bradley:

> *"[...I]t would be the fate of every person to be decimated every year of his life in order to know whether he would have smallpox this year or not, right up to the moment when that fate actually befell him."*

What Bernoulli referred to can be understood mathematically referring to the following expression:

$$\Pr(x = j) = \left(1 - \frac{1}{n}\right)^{j-1} \frac{1}{n},$$

where x is the year during which smallpox will be acquired. The term $(1 - \frac{1}{n})$ represents the "escape probability" q during one year. If a person escapes infec-

[2] In the original: "*... deux articles cu'on ne connoît que fort superficiellement.*" (Last sentence of §2)

[3] *[...] le sort de chaque personne seroit d'être décimée chaque année de sa vie, pour savoir si elle aura cette même année la petite vérole ou non, jusqu'à ce que le sort fût tomebé une fois sur elle.*

tion until year j, then q has to be multiplied $j-1$ times (the number of years infection is escaped). Therefore, q is raised to the $(j-1)$th power. For the year during which infection will take place, that term is multiplied by the annual probability of infection, $\frac{1}{n}$. Clearly, $\Pr(x)$ is a declining function of x, as can easily be verified, which supports Bernoulli's statement.

The revolutionary insight manifesting here is that the declining incidence of smallpox by age was not driven by declining susceptibility, but rather by a depletion of the number of individuals still available for infection. In paragraph §4, Bernoulli mentions and justifies the use of the mortality table constructed by Edmond Halley (1656 to 1742) as a basis for his own calculations. These tables, apparently, were based on observations from Breslaw, but seem to have been "amended" by smoothing out irregularities, in order to achieve "uniformity of law in variations".[4] He discusses his choice of the size of the fictional birth cohort being 1300; Halley's list begins with the numbers alive after the first year.

1.1.2 §5 through §6: Mathematical foundation

Paragraphs §5 and §6 develop the mathematical foundation for the tools used to answer the key question: "What is the gain of inoculation?". The argument is relatively simple. Let me start with a list of the most important symbols:

- x is the age in years; as we are dealing with a birth cohort born at the same time, x can be treated as time;
- ξ is the number surviving to a certain age;
- s is the number not yet having had smallpox (and thus still susceptible) at a given age;
- $\frac{1}{n}$ is the annual smallpox attack rate in people not yet having had smallpox and who thus are still susceptible;
- $\frac{1}{m}$ is the case fatality ratio for smallpox.

The goal is to express s as a function of x, ξ, n, and m. Let ds denote the change—always decrease—in the number of susceptible to smallpox in the infinitesimally small time interval dx. As ds must be negative, $-ds$ represents the number of smallpox infections during that time interval. As this number is a real number and not an integer, it might be more accurate to refer to the "amount" of smallpox infections. Also, if mortality due to other causes is ignored first,

$$-ds = \frac{sdx}{n} \tag{1.1}$$

because $\frac{1}{n}$ is the annual risk of infection of a susceptible individual; there are s susceptible individuals (multiply) and the time is an infinitesimal fraction of a year (dx; multiply). The negative sign is necessary because ds is, intrinsically, negative: The birth cohort can only dwindle. The right-hand side of expression (1.1), on the other hand, is intrinsically positive.

[4] *[...] uniformité del loi dans les variations.*

Question 1.c

The infectious process in Bernoulli's model is driven by the annual "attack rate" $\frac{1}{n}$ ("over the course of a year, out of n persons, one will acquire smallpox"). Is there a conflict between this definition and the use of the parameter n or rather $\frac{1}{n}$ in Eq. (1.1)?

The number of those dying from smallpox during dx accordingly can be written as $\frac{sdx}{nm}$, by multiplying the number of new infections, $\frac{sdx}{n}$, with the case fatality ratio, $\frac{1}{m}$. The total number dying of any cause during infinitesimal time interval dx is $-d\xi$ because ξ can only decrease (the birth cohort cannot be augmented!) and therefore $d\xi$ is intrinsically negative. Then, the number dying of other causes than smallpox during interval dx is given by $-d\xi - \frac{sdx}{nm}$, i.e. from all deaths ($-d\xi$) the deaths due to smallpox have to be subtracted. The negative signs tend to be confusing at first![5] The following substitution will help the confusion:

$$du = -d\xi - \frac{sdx}{nm}, \tag{1.2}$$

i.e. u represents the deaths due to causes other than smallpox. The following equation results:

$$-ds = \frac{sdx}{n} + du\frac{s}{\xi}. \tag{1.3}$$

The final fraction in expression (1.3) is justified by the assertion that the number of susceptible does not only decrease due to smallpox infection,[6] but also by mortality due to other causes; that, however, matters only in the susceptible portion of the population. Therefore, du is multiplied by the proportion of susceptible in the population, $\frac{s}{\xi}$.

Substituting the expression (1.2) for du into Eq. (1.3), we arrive at Bernoulli's key expression:

$$\begin{aligned} -ds &= \frac{sdx}{n} + \left(-d\xi - \frac{sdx}{nm}\right)\frac{s}{\xi} \\ &= \frac{sdx}{n} - \frac{sd\xi}{\xi} - \frac{ssdx}{nm\xi}. \end{aligned} \tag{1.4}$$

Question 1.d

What does Eq. (1.4) imply for the relationship between smallpox and mortality due to other causes? Is this assumption reasonable?

[5] When reading this passage in Bradley's translation first, I thought there was a transcription error.

[6] It is, by the way, irrelevant for the present calculation if people infected by smallpox die or not; either way they lose their susceptibility!

Manipulating expression (1.4) we obtain

$$\frac{sd\xi}{\xi} - ds = \frac{sdx}{n} - \frac{s^2dx}{nm}$$

which, after multiplying by $\frac{\xi}{s^2}$, becomes

$$\frac{sd\xi - ds\xi}{s^2} = \frac{\xi dx}{sn} - \frac{dx}{nm\xi}. \tag{1.5}$$

Bernoulli then lets $q = \frac{\xi}{s}$ which, when substituted into Eq. (1.5), gives

$$dq = \frac{qdx}{n} - \frac{dx}{nm}, \tag{1.6}$$

which, after multiplying both sides with nm, yields

$$mndq = mqdx - dx, \tag{1.7}$$

and, finally, algebraically manipulating, dividing both sides by dx,

$$\begin{aligned} \frac{mndq}{dx} &= mq - 1, \\ \frac{mndq}{mq-1} &= dx, \\ dx &= \frac{mndq}{mq-1}, \\ dx &= \frac{mn}{mq-1}dq. \end{aligned} \tag{1.8}$$

Integrating expression (1.8) results in

$$\int dx = \int \frac{mn}{mq-1}dq, \tag{1.9}$$

$$x + C = n\ln(mq-1) \tag{1.10}$$

$$= n\ln\left(\frac{m\xi}{s} - 1\right). \tag{1.11}$$

Comment on Eqs. (1.9)–(1.11)

The integral on the right-hand side in (1.9) is computed by first factoring n (a constant), letting $u = mq - 1$ and $du = mdq$. The latter expression is true because $du = \frac{du}{dq}dq$ and the derivative of $umq - 1$ with respect to q is m. Therefore, $du = mdq$. Further, $\int \frac{mn}{mq-1}dq$ thus can be rewritten as $n\int \frac{1}{u}dq$ which, according to fundamental rules of integration, is $n\ln(u) + C$, C being the constant of integration and, substituting for u, $n\ln(mq-1) + C$.

Expression (1.11) can be transformed and exponentiated on both sides to give

$$\begin{aligned} x + C &= n \ln\left(\frac{m\xi}{s} - 1\right), \\ \exp(x + C) &= \left(\frac{m\xi}{s} - 1\right)^n, \\ \exp\left(\frac{x + C}{n}\right) &= \left(\frac{m\xi}{s} - 1\right), \qquad (1.12) \\ s &= \frac{m\xi}{\exp(\frac{x+C}{n}) + 1}. \qquad (1.13) \end{aligned}$$

Finally, the initial condition problem has to be solved: At birth, when $x = 0$, everybody is susceptible, i.e. $\xi = s$ and $\frac{\xi}{s} = 1$, changing Eq. (1.12) to

$$\exp\left(\frac{C}{n}\right) = m - 1.$$

Now, if Eq. (1.12) is used in expression (1.13), we arrive at the final formula that is used to create the two tables in the back of the article:

$$\begin{aligned} s &= \frac{m\xi}{\exp(\frac{x+C}{n}) + 1} \\ &= \frac{m\xi}{(m-1)\exp(\frac{x}{n}) + 1} \\ &= \frac{8\xi}{7\exp(\frac{x}{7}) + 1}. \qquad (1.14) \end{aligned}$$

The latter equation is completed by plugging in the assumed values of n and m.

1.1.3 §7 through §9: Table 1

In §7, Bernoulli gives a detailed explanation of the first table at the end of the article that follows a virtual cohort of 1,300 newborn. The following Table 1.1 is a reproduction of Table 1. The values were calculated using Bernoulli's method, but with a few small computational errors corrected. The calculations were done in a spreadsheet program (see online material). As opposed to us, Bernoulli could not take advantage of automated computation!

First column Age or time x which is equivalent as the members of the cohort are of same age.

Second column Survivors ξ at year x. $\xi(2)$, e.g. would be the survivors at the end of the second year (i.e. when they turn 2). This is observable.

Third column Those not having had smallpox, s at time x. This number is calculated using formula (1.14), using the first two columns as input.

Fourth column The number of those having acquired smallpox during year x is calculated as the difference between all survivors in column 2 ($\xi(x)$) and those who have not yet had smallpox in column 3 ($s(x)$).

Table 1.1 **This is the first of the two tables, slightly modified from the original, with some computational errors corrected**

Age in years	Surviving according Mr. Halley	Not having had smallpox	Having had smallpox	Acquiring smallpox each year	Deaths from smallpox each year	Sum of smallpox deaths	Deaths of other causes each year
0	1300	1300	0				
1	1000	896	104	137	17.1	17.1	283
2	855	685	170	99	12.4	29.5	133
3	798	571	227	79	9.9	39.4	47
4	760	485	275	66	8.3	47.7	30
5	732	416	316	56	7	54.7	21
6	710	359	351	48	6	60.7	16
7	692	311	381	42	5.3	66	12.7
8	680	272	408	36	4.5	70.5	7.5
9	670	238	432	32	4	74.5	6
10	661	208	453	28	3.5	78	5.5
11	653	182	471	24.4	3.1	81.1	4.9
12	646	160	486	21.4	2.7	83.8	4.3
13	640	140	500	18.7	2.4	86.2	3.6
14	634	123	511	16.6	2.1	88.3	3.9
15	628	108	520	14.4	1.8	90.1	4.2
16	622	94	528	12.6	1.6	91.7	4.4
17	616	83	533	11.0	1.4	93.1	4.6
18	610	72	538	9.7	1.2	94.3	4.8
19	604	63	541	8.4	1.1	95.4	4.9
20	598	55	543	7.4	0.9	96.3	5.1
21	592	48.5	543.5	6.5	0.8	97.1	5.2
22	586	42.4	543.6	5.6	0.7	97.8	5.3
23	579	37	542	5	0.6	98.4	6.4
24	572	32.3	539.7	4.4	0.5	98.9	6.5

Fifth column This column contains the "imputed"[7] number of people having caught smallpox at time/age x. Realizing that the pool of susceptible would be diminished over the course of a year, by both infection and non-smallpox mortality, he proposed to average the survivor data for time x and $x - 1$.

Question 1.e

Discuss limitations for the described averaging approach.

Sixth column This column consists of those having died from smallpox and is obtained by multiplying the fifth column (all those having acquired smallpox during that year) by the case fatality ratio $\frac{1}{m}$ with $m = 8$.

Seventh column This column contains the cumulative sum of smallpox victims.

Eighth column The final column lists the annual number of deaths due to other causes and is calculated by subtracting the number having died of smallpox (column 6) from the total number having died in year x, $\xi(x-1) - \xi(x)$ for $x > 0$.

Question 1.f

Why did I, at the beginning of the chapter, qualify Bradley's statement "[...] first attempt at a mathematical theory of the propagation of an infectious disease" as inaccurate?

Comment on possible discrepancy

In §8, Bernoulli comments on the fact that Table 1 which "perfectly conforms to our hypotheses" does not exactly reflect "nature". He mentions the number of 137 children who, according to the Table, acquire smallpox during their first year, but that this number appears to be quite large. Nevertheless, he advises not to discard these numbers without new evidence. It is actually likely that the number of small children suffering from smallpox was smaller than Bernoulli's model predicted because of maternal antibodies that protected them for six months or so.

Further observations

Under §9, Bernoulli then comments in great detail on his observations in Table 1, listing items *(a)* through *(o)*. I list here only a few:

(a) Being a little more than six years of age, half of the surviving children have had smallpox; at 15 years, only about a sixth of the surviving have been spared, and by the age of 24 it is only $\frac{1}{18}$. In fact, the chance of a newborn to suffer from smallpox *or* die before the age of 24 is 39 to 1 (97.5%).

(c) Up to and including age 24, 101 persons of the cohort of size 1,300 will die from smallpox, which is about $\frac{1}{13}$.

[7] The term "imputed" has been set in quotes because imputation is more meaningfully used in the context of real data; here, the data is artificial.

(d) Half of the deaths from smallpox occur before the age of five.
(e) If it were not for smallpox, the ages of 12 and 13 would be the "most secure age" (*l'année la plus sûre*).
(m) If we think of the continuous succession and coexistence of birth cohorts of 1,300, the annual number of smallpox cases is 800 (number provided by Bernoulli); consulting the Table of the spreadsheet we calculate 790 by adding up column 5: The annual contribution of each birth cohort is just the number corresponding to the age-specific numbers of smallpox cases. Bernoulli thus calculates the average number of smallpox cases for Paris, where approximately 18 thousand children were born each year during his time. That is, given a birth cohort size of 18,000, 11,000 smallpox cases would result each year and, assuming a duration of illness of one month, the number 900 is obtained.

1.1.4 §11 & §12: Table 2

The second table presents the key findings of this analysis that represent an answer to the question: "What would be the impact of universal inoculation?"

Table 2 (here Table 1.2) is represented here, again with small numerical deviations from Bernoulli's table. The values were calculated exactly as prescribed by Bernoulli to obtain the *counterfactual*[8] number of survivors each year as follows:

1. If smallpox is eliminated as a cause of death, mortality can only occur from death "due to other causes". Assuming that that mortality is the same in the population *not* affected by smallpox, we can estimate the respective rate from Table 1:
   a. During the first year, there are, in the natural state, 17.1 deaths due to smallpox. These deaths would not occur in the smallpox-free state. Therefore, at the beginning of the next year, there would be 1017.1 instead of 1000 survivors.
   b. To compute the counterfactual numbers of deaths in the smallpox-free world, the observed mortality due to non-smallpox causes, which is in Bernoulli's notation

$$\frac{r}{q},$$

   where r is the number of non-smallpox deaths (eighth column of Table 1: 133) and q is the number of survivors at the beginning of that age-year, in the "natural" state (column 2, Table 1: 1,000).
2. This rate would have to be applied to the *new* number of people at risk, here 1017.1. This gives 135.3 deaths.
3. To obtain the counterfactual numbers surviving at the beginning of the next year, the number of deaths (135.3) has to be subtracted from the number of those that had survived to the beginning of the current year (1117.1), giving 881.8.

These calculations are repeated to the desired age. Note that the last row of Table 2, for age 25, cannot be calculated from Table 1 which only provides data for calculating

[8] A *counterfactual* quantity refers to a quantity which is not observable, but represents an observed quantity under different circumstances; here, under the absence of smallpox.

Table 1.2 **The following caption, translated from French, is given for this Table 2: "This Table makes apparent, how may of 1,300 children, assumed to be borne at the same time, remain alive from year to year until the age of 25 if one assumes that all are exposed to smallpox; and how many would remain if all were freed from that disease, with the comparison and difference of these two states." Again, a few numerical errors were corrected; there is a typo in the original table: The counterfactual number of survivors at age 13 should be 714.4 instead of 741.1—the survivors can never *increase* with increasing age! The numbers were calculated using Bernoulli's method and a spreadsheet program (see online supplement)**

Age in years	Survivors, natural state	Survivors, no smallpox	Difference
0	1300	1300	0
1	1000	1017.1	17.1
2	855	881.8	26.8
3	798	833.3	35.3
4	760	802	42
5	732	779.8	47.8
6	710	762.8	52.8
7	692	749.2	57.2
8	680	741.1	61.1
9	670	734.6	64.6
10	661	728.6	67.6
11	653	723.2	70.2
12	646	718.4	72.4
13	640	714.4	74.4
14	634	710	76
15	628	705.3	77.3
16	622	700.4	78.4
17	616	695.2	79.2
18	610	689.8	79.8
19	604	684.3	80.3
20	598	678.5	80.5
21	592	672.6	80.6
22	586	666.6	80.6
23	579	659.3	80.3
24	572	651.9	79.9
25	565	644.4	79.4

the counterfactual number alive to age 24. I therefore used the number of deaths from the previous age-year to calculate the counterfactual number alive (number off by 0.1 from Bernoulli's number).

The question Bernoulli set out to study concerned the gain due to effectively eliminating smallpox mortality by the use of *inoculation*. That gain, up to age 25, can be seen in the last row of Table 2 and is 79.4—this represents the difference in survivors between the counterfactual, smallpox-free, and the natural state.

Question 1.g

Is the difference in the last row of Table 2 a good representation of the gain due to inoculation?

Bernoulli discusses the problem of how to quantify the gain due to inoculation in great detail. This discussion may be of particular interest to those interested in demography. But I need to point out his approach to compute the "total quantity of life" (*quantité de vie totale*) and from that derive the *average live* (= life expectancy). The methods are straightforward and the interested reader is encouraged to peruse these passages (§12, (f)). Briefly, the annual survival numbers are added for both states, with a correction applied to account for the fact that mortality is distributed throughout the year, and divided by the cohort size (1,300). The result of these calculations is quite impressive:

Bernoulli calculated the life expectancy for the **natural state as 26 years and 7 months**; for the counterfactual, **smallpox mortality-free state that number is 29 years and 9 months**; the gain in life expectancy being about **two seventeenths ($\frac{2}{17}$) of the natural life expectancy**.

1.1.5 §13: Closed form solution for the counterfactual survivors

I will conclude this chapter with a brief description of Bernoulli's derivation for the counterfactual numbers of survivors, or, to be exact, for the ratio of the numbers corresponding to the new states.

1. Let ζ denote the number of survivors in the counterfactual state without smallpox mortality. As we have seen before, $-d\xi$ represents the total mortality during the infinitesimal age interval dx.
2. The mortality without smallpox is that number with the smallpox mortality subtracted,

$$-\xi - \frac{sdx}{mn}.$$

3. To scale that to the counterfactual survivors, this quantity is multiplied by $\frac{\zeta}{\xi}$ which then describes the mortality in the counterfactual state, $-d\zeta$, i.e.

$$-d\zeta \quad = \quad -\frac{\zeta}{\xi}\left(d\xi + \frac{sdx}{mn}\right),$$

$$\frac{d\zeta}{\zeta} - \frac{d\xi}{\xi} = \frac{\frac{1}{n}dx}{(m-1)e^{\frac{x}{n}} + 1} \tag{1.15}$$

(substituting for s using (1.14)).

4. Integrating both sides of (1.15), using the "common rules" (*les règles connues*):

$$\frac{\zeta}{\xi} = \frac{me^{\frac{1}{n}}}{(m-1)e^{\frac{x}{n}} + 1}. \tag{1.16}$$

Question 1.h

It is quite possible that Bernoulli was fluent regarding the rules of integration. I personally, however, find how the "common rules" apply here not all that obvious. Is it obvious to you? Can you derive Eq. (1.16)?

Bernoulli comments on the superior precision of numbers resulting from applying this formula rather than using the approximation on which Table 2 is based, but we are leaving it at that.

Appendix 1.A Answers

1.a First, to be more precise, let $d_s(\tau)$ and $d_T(\tau)$ denote the cumulative numbers of deaths due to smallpox and in total, respectively from time $t = 0$ up to time $t = \tau$. If that time interval is very long, the ratio will approach the average probability P_s at birth for a randomly picked individual born in that interval to die from smallpox. This could be expressed as

$$\lim_{\tau \to \infty} \frac{d_s(\tau)}{d_T(\tau)} = P_s.$$

If that probability, which can be interpreted as a proportional mortality ratio, holds for an individual, it must also hold for a "generation". The term "generation" refers to a cohort of people born at a given day, in a given week, month, year, or decade. If the risk to die from smallpox were to be very different just outside of the interval $(0, \tau]$ than within, then $\frac{d_s(t)}{d_T(t)} \neq P_s$: For the sake of the argument, assume that the risk to die of smallpox is μ_s for times $t > \tau$, but 0 for $t \in (0, \tau]$. Accordingly, $d_s(\tau) = 0$ and thus $P_s(\tau) = 0$ even though, for any individual born after time τ the risk to die from smallpox would be greater than 0. Clearly, the longer the interval τ, the smaller the influence of such potential bias. However, if the population under investigation is undergoing substantial demographic changes, further bias could be introduced (why?). Despite these issues, the answer to this question would likely be a qualified "yes", indicating that the ratio of smallpox deaths to all deaths reasonably represents the proportionate mortality ratio for smallpox under a wide range of assumptions.

1.b Bernoulli's belief that observing a very long time series of cause-specific mortality in many different populations would be informative as to the "natural constant" of smallpox mortality risk is, from today's perspective, misguided. Infectious disease risk is not a natural constant: This is at the very core of infectious disease epidemiology and will, in one way or the other, follow us throughout this book.

1.c The use of the annual attack rate $AR = \frac{1}{n}$ in Eq. (1.1) is problematic because the attack rate represents a probability while the term $\frac{1}{n}$ in the equation represents a rate. As an extreme example one could imagine a situation in which the annual attack rate is very high, say $AR = 0.99$. The corresponding annual incidence rate is 4.60517. This can be shown as follows (if you are familiar with important features of the exponential distribution, skip the following text box):

Exponential distribution

The exponential distribution is defined as

$$f(t) = \lambda e^{-\lambda t},$$

where $f(t)$ represents the probability density of the *failure times*; these are the times when the first event occurs, when the rate of occurrence is λ. One reason for the great epidemiological importance of the exponential distribution lies in the relationship between the "failure" or, similarly, the "survival" probability. Failure and survival in this case refer to the occurrence (= failure) of non-occurrence (= survival) of such an event. The failure probability $P_f(t)$ for a particular time period (e.g. from 0 to t) can be expressed as the probability that the event occurs at time t or before. Mathematically, this can be expressed as

$$\begin{aligned} P_f(t) &= \int_{u=0}^{t} \lambda e^{-\lambda u} du \\ &= 1 - e^{-\lambda t}. \end{aligned}$$

The survival probability is the complement of $P_f(t)$, i.e. $P_s(t) = 1 - P_f(t)$. The exponential distribution is closely associated with the Poisson distribution which characterizes the probability distribution of the number of events occurring in a given time period given a rate.

The AR corresponds to the $P_f(t) = 0.99$. As we know that $P_f(t) = 1 - e^{-\lambda t}$ we can solve that expression for λ:

- First, write $0.99 = 1 - e^{-\lambda t}$.
- Second, by rearranging, rewrite as $e^{-\lambda t} = 1 - 0.99$.
- Finally, take the logarithm of both sides and multiply both sides by -1, which gives $\lambda t = -\log(0.01) = 4.60517$.

Note that λt represents the annual "failure rate"; λ could represent an annual rate and $t = 1$ (year), or a daily rate, and $t = 365$ (days), etc. If that rate is doubled, the annual attack rate only changes marginally to $1 - e^{-4.60517 \times 2} = 0.9999$. If the rate and the corresponding attack rate are small, say $P_f(t) = 0.01$, then we can write $P_f(t) \approx \lambda t$ and the problem pointed out becomes negligible. (Try it with a calculator or calculating software!)

1.d Expression (1.4) assumes total mortality from other causes than smallpox that is stated by Eq. (1.2) (total mortality at age x minus smallpox mortality at that age). The fraction $\frac{s}{\xi}$ implies that the non-smallpox mortality applied to the proportion of susceptible is valid; this implies that the non-smallpox mortality is the same in those immune to smallpox and thus that smallpox and non-smallpox mortality are independent. It is possible to think of situations where that may not be true, but it appears to be a reasonable assumption.

1.e The procedure Bernoulli implements seems intuitively reasonable: If the expected number of cases x needs to be calculated, produced by an incidence rate, say λ, that acts on a particular amount of "person-time", say τ, then we simply multiply the rate with the person-time, $E(x) = \lambda \times \tau$. If you are unfamiliar with the epidemiological concept of person-time at risk, this quantity is defined as the total time "contributed" by all members of a group/population during which an event of interest (e.g. smallpox infection) could have happened. In the case of smallpox, only susceptible persons would contribute person-time.
Now we know the incidence rate ($\frac{1}{N}$ per person per year). But what about the person-time? We know the number of susceptibles at the beginning of each year of life. But that number will decline during the year due to smallpox infection and mortality from other cases.
Assuming that the rates remain constant during a year (smallpox incidence and non-smallpox mortality) the susceptible will actually decline exponentially. This is illustrated in Fig. 1.1.
The gray area could have been calculated by solving the function (using the numbers from the Table) for $\lambda : \frac{896}{1,300} = \exp(-\lambda t)$ where $t = 1$ (one year) and then integrating the function.
But to make a long story short, Bernoulli's approach was a reasonable approximation; even in the quite extreme example ($\lambda = 0.5$, which is a substantial rate) the error (orange segment) is small.

1.f The answer would be much more obvious further into this book: While Bernoulli's paper was clearly highly original and a pioneering work of epidemiology and demographics, it does not deal with the dynamic aspect of transmission. Rather, it treats the incidence of infection as a constant. As we will see, the fact that the risk of infection is a function of the intensity of transmission is the fundamental reason why transmission modeling is so interesting and necessary.

1.g The problem is most obvious when we construct a hypothetical extension to Table 2 that reaches to the age of, say 130. At that point, of course, there would not be any difference any more because everybody would have already died, i.e. no survivors in either the natural or the counterfactual state. Even though the difference in surviving subjects at a relatively young age when most would have already acquired smallpox is a good indicator of benefit of inoculation it cannot be used as a straightforward measure of gain.

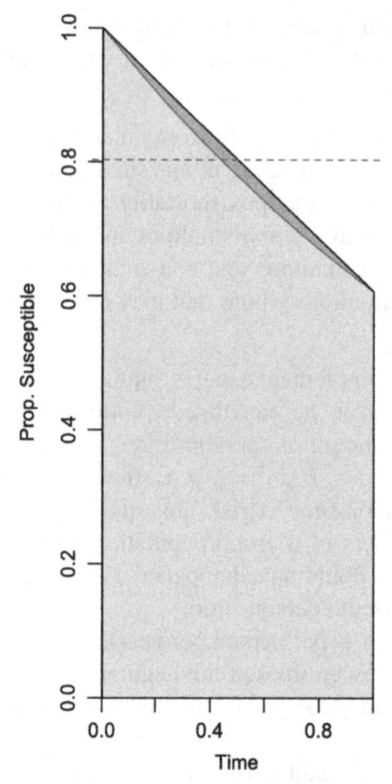

Figure 1.1 This is a hypothetical example. The light gray area represents the correct proportion susceptible. The light gray plus the dark gray (orange in the online figure) area corresponds to the person-time obtained by Bernoulli's approach; the average is shown with the dashed (red) line.

1.h The question here is, how do we get from (1.15), that is,

$$\frac{d\zeta}{\zeta} - \frac{d\xi}{\xi} = \frac{\frac{1}{n}dx}{(m-1)e^{\frac{x}{n}} + 1},$$

to (1.16), namely

$$\frac{\zeta}{\xi} = \frac{me^{\frac{1}{n}}}{(m-1)e^{\frac{x}{n}} + 1}?$$

There are several steps involved, but the left-hand side is relatively easy to deal with. It involves the two fractions $\frac{d\zeta}{\zeta}$ and $\frac{d\xi}{\xi}$; both are handled exactly the same way, using the basic rules of integration. So if we integrate the first fraction, from age 0 ($x = 0$) to age x_1, we get

$$\begin{aligned}\int_{x=0}^{x_1} \frac{d\zeta}{\zeta} &= \int \frac{1}{\zeta}\, d\zeta \\ &= \log|\zeta|\Big|_0^{x_1} \\ &= \log \zeta(x_1) - \log(\zeta(0)). \end{aligned} \tag{1.17}$$

By the way, the basic rule of integration applied here can relatively easily be derived, but I will not do that here. We will not leave the vertical bars off because we are dealing with strictly positive quantities. Applying the same to the second fraction, we get

$$\int_{x=0}^{x_1} \frac{d\xi}{\xi} = \log \xi(x_1) - \log(\xi(0)). \tag{1.18}$$

The left-hand side of (1.15) therefore becomes, after integration,

$$\begin{aligned}&(\log \zeta(x_1) - \log(\zeta(0))) - (\log \xi(x_1) - \log(\xi(0))) \\ &= \log \zeta(x_1) - \log(\zeta(0)) - \log \xi(x_1) + \log(\xi(0)) \\ &= \log \zeta(x_1) - \log \xi(x_1) \text{ (see comment below)} \\ &= \log \frac{\zeta(x_1)}{\xi(x_1)} \text{ (use property of log to rewrite).}\end{aligned} \tag{1.19}$$

The $\zeta(0)$ and $\xi(0)$ "cancel" because at age 0, regardless of whether smallpox mortality is high or not, the numbers of surviving are equal and thus the difference is 0. We might, of course, think of situations where that may not be the case, but here we assume that birth rates and thus the resulting *birth cohorts* are unaffected by smallpox. The right-hand side of (1.19) is due to the fact that the difference of logarithms of two functions equals the logarithm of the *fraction* of the two functions.

The integration of the right-hand side of (1.15) is a little more difficult to tackle and requires the following four steps:

1. We apply *u substitution* to the expression

$$\frac{\frac{1}{n}dx}{(m-1)e^{\frac{x}{n}}+1}.$$

The principle of u substitution is the following: If we have an integral like $\int f(x)dx$, we would like to rewrite it as follows

$$\int f(x)dx = \int g(u)du \tag{1.20}$$

if the integral on the right-hand side can be more easily computed. Note that

$$du = u'dx = \frac{du}{dx}dx. \tag{1.21}$$

In our case, we can accomplish this as follows:

$$\begin{aligned}
\frac{\frac{1}{n}dx}{(m-1)e^{\frac{x}{n}}+1} &= \frac{\frac{1}{n}e^{\frac{x}{n}}dx}{(m-1)\left(e^{\frac{x}{n}}\right)^2+e^{\frac{x}{n}}} \\
&\quad \text{(multiply numerator and denominator by } e^{\frac{x}{n}}\text{)} \\
&= \frac{\frac{1}{n}udx}{(m-1)u^2+u} \text{ (call } u=e^{\frac{x}{n}}\text{)} \\
&= \frac{du}{(m-1)u^2+u} \text{ (see explanation below).} \qquad (1.22)
\end{aligned}$$

A brief remark on the substitution $\frac{1}{n}udx = du$: Now if we plug-in what u actually is and note that the derivative of $e^{\frac{x}{n}}$ with respect to x is $\frac{1}{n}e^{\frac{x}{n}}$, we get

$$\frac{1}{n}e^{\frac{x}{n}}dx = \frac{de^{\frac{x}{n}}}{dx}dx = de^{\frac{x}{n}} = du. \qquad (1.23)$$

2. Now we have the somewhat simplified form of the right-hand side of (1.15), but we have more work to do. If we look at the fraction

$$\frac{du}{(m-1)u^2+u},$$

you may or may not realize that a partial fraction decomposition is what we need to bring the integral into a "bite-sized" form. I will demonstrate the steps:

$$\begin{aligned}
\frac{1}{(m-1)u^2+u} &= \frac{1}{u\left((m-1)u+1\right)} \qquad (1.24) \\
&= \frac{A}{u}+\frac{B}{(m-1)u+1} \qquad (1.25) \\
&\quad \text{(this is what we would like to get, but do not know } A, B\text{)} \\
&= \frac{1}{u}-\frac{k}{ku+1} \qquad (1.26) \\
&\quad \text{(letting } k=m-1\text{—see explanation that follows).}
\end{aligned}$$

To get from the right-hand side of (1.24) to (1.26), we needed to solve for A and B. To do this, we multiply both sides of

$$\frac{1}{u\,(ku+1)} = \frac{A}{u}+\frac{B}{ku+1} \qquad (1.27)$$

by the common denominator, $u\,(ku+1)$, to get

$$\begin{aligned}
\frac{u\,(ku+1)}{u\,(ku+1)} &= \frac{A\,u\,(ku+1)}{u}+\frac{B\,u\,(ku+1)}{ku+1}, \\
1 &= A\,(ku+1)+B\,u \text{ (denominators cancel).} \qquad (1.28)
\end{aligned}$$

Eq. (1.28) can be solved for A and B: First, set $u = 0$; we can do this, as the relationship described by (1.28) must hold for any value of u. This gives

$$\begin{aligned} 1 &= A\,(k0+1)+B0 \\ &= A \text{ (solution for } A=1). \end{aligned} \tag{1.29}$$

Now do the same process for B, setting $ku = -1$ so that A vanishes; u must then be $u = -\frac{1}{k}$:

$$\begin{aligned} 1 &= A\left(k\left(-\frac{1}{k}\right)+1\right)+B\left(-\frac{1}{k}\right) \\ &= -\frac{B}{k} \text{ (the term with } A \text{ vanishes)}, \\ B &= -k \text{ (solution for } B \text{ after rearranging)}. \end{aligned} \tag{1.30}$$

3. Now we have to compute the integral of the right-hand side of (1.26) with respect to u:

$$\begin{aligned} \int \frac{1}{u} - \frac{k}{ku+1} du &= \int \frac{1}{u} du - \int \frac{k}{ku+1} du \\ &= \int \frac{1}{u} du - \int \frac{k}{ku+1} du \\ &= \log|u| - \log|ku+1| \\ &= \log|e^{\frac{x}{n}}| - \log|(m-1)e^{\frac{x}{n}}+1| \\ &\quad \text{(resubstituting } u \text{ with } e^{\frac{x}{n}} \text{ and } k \text{ with } m-1) \\ \int \frac{\frac{1}{n}}{(m-1)e^{\frac{x}{n}}+1} dx &= \log \frac{e^{\frac{x}{n}}}{(m-1)e^{\frac{x}{n}}+1} \\ &\quad \text{(again using } \log a - \log b = \log \frac{a}{b}). \end{aligned} \tag{1.31}$$

For the left-hand side of Eq. (1.31) I used the integral of the right-hand side of Eq. (1.15) which we set out to integrate. To complete this step, though, we have to compute the definite integral of the right-hand side of Eq. (1.15), i.e. from age $x = 0$ to age $x = x_1$:

$$\int_0^{x_1} \frac{\frac{1}{n}}{(m-1)e^{\frac{x}{n}}+1} dx.$$

This is not difficult to accomplish using our results:

$$\begin{aligned} \int_0^{x_1} \frac{\frac{1}{n}}{(m-1)e^{\frac{x}{n}}+1} dx &= \log \frac{e^{\frac{x}{n}}}{(m-1)e^{\frac{x}{n}}+1}\Bigg|_0^{x_1} \\ &= \log \frac{e^{\frac{x_1}{n}}}{(m-1)e^{\frac{x_1}{n}}+1} - \log \frac{e^{\frac{0}{n}}}{(m-1)e^{\frac{0}{n}}+1} \end{aligned}$$

$$
\begin{aligned}
&= \log \frac{e^{\frac{x_1}{n}}}{(m-1)e^{\frac{x_1}{n}}+1} - \log \frac{1}{m} \\
&\quad (e^{\frac{0}{n}} = 1 \text{ in numerator and denominator}) \\
&= \log \frac{m\, e^{\frac{x_1}{n}}}{(m-1)e^{\frac{x_1}{n}}+1} \qquad (1.32) \\
&\quad \left(\text{using } \log C - \log \frac{1}{m} = \log \frac{C}{\frac{1}{m}} = \log m\, C\right).
\end{aligned}
$$

4. Putting (1.19) and (1.32) together, we get

$$
\log \frac{\zeta(x_1)}{\xi(x_1)} = \log \left(\frac{m\, e^{\frac{x_1}{n}}}{(m-1)e^{\frac{x_1}{n}}+1} \right). \qquad (1.33)
$$

Exponentiating both sides of Eq. (1.33), we obtain Eq. (1.16) and have thus answered the question.

Appendix 1.B Supplementary material

Supplementary material related to this chapter can be found online at http://dx.doi.org/10.1016/B978-0-12-802260-3.00001-8.

References

[1] D. Bernoulli, Essai d'une nouvelle analyse de la mortalité causée par lat petite Vérole, & des avantages de l'inoculation pour la prévenir, 1760.

[2] D. Bernoulli, S. Blower, An attempt at a new analysis of the mortality caused by smallpox and of the advantages of inoculation to prevent it, Reviews in Medical Virology 14 (5) (2004) 275–288, Wiley Online Library.

[3] L. Bradley, Smallpox Inoculation: An Eighteenth Century Mathematical Controversy: Translation and Critical Commentary by L. Bradley, University of Nottingham, Dept. of Adult Education [Matlock], ISBN 0902031236, 1971.

[4] K. Dietz, J. Heesterbeek, Bernoulli was ahead of modern epidemiology, Nature 408 (6812) (2000) 513–514.

[5] K. Dietz, J. Heesterbeek, Daniel Bernoulli's epidemiological model revisited, Mathematical Biosciences 180 (1) (2002) 1–21.

P.D. En'ko: An early transmission model (1889)

2

Contents

2.1 Introduction

Like many absolute statements on the historic evolution of transmission models, the assertion that the object of this chapter, P.D. En'ko's paper [1], is the first "true" description of a transmission model is of uncertain truth. But quite certainly, it is one of the first and would not have come to my attention had Klaus Dietz not translated the Russian paper into English and republished it in the International Journal of Epidemiology.

En'ko develops a transmission model, basically from "first principles", i.e. based on some specific assumptions, but without resorting to previously developed theory. He then compares "synthetic epidemics" the numbers of which are calculated using the model to actual outbreaks of measles and scarlet fever in two boarding schools, the *Imperial Educational College for the Daughters of the Nobility* and the *Alexander Institution*, a "School for the Daughters of Burghers" in St Petersburg between 1875 and 1888. We will largely limit our discussion on measles. Of note, the bacterial etiology of scarlet fever was known at the time of publication of En'ko's paper, but whether he was aware of this is unclear. That measles was caused by an infectious agent was also well-known; however, the existence of viruses had not yet been established.

2.2 Assumptions

The assumptions that form the basis for En'ko's transmission model are quite straightforward:

A Historical Introduction to Mathematical Modeling of Infectious Diseases. DOI: 10.1016/B978-0-12-802260-3.00002-X

1. All susceptibles are fully susceptible.
2. All immunes are completely immune.
3. The probability of becoming infected equals the probability of coming in contact with a case during one period.
4. The population is of size N with J being susceptible and x are infected; these are all variables. This is also true for N: as the ill get transferred to the infirmary, the population N decreases.
5. If x people become infected/infectious during period t they will be capable of infecting others during period $t+1$ after which they will be removed from the population: This paper deals with outbreaks in boarding schools; sick are transferred to the infirmary.
6. A is what we will call the transmission parameter, even though it is introduced by En'ko as follows:

   > *"A is the number of contacts of ill people with healthy individuals." (p. 750, first column, second paragraph)*

   Considering expression (2.3) below, as we will do, the interpretation of A as transmission parameter, or more specifically, will become clear.
7. The number of potentially infectious contacts A is proportional to the size of the population so that A/N is constant.
8. An implicit assumption is that the probabilities of coming in contact with any other member in the population are the same.

2.3 The model

From these assumptions it follows that the probability of getting in contact with an infected when meeting a person is $\frac{x}{N-1}$.

Question 2.a

Why is the denominator of this expression $N-1$?

The probability of not coming in contact with one of the x infecteds[1] is the complement, i.e.

$$\begin{aligned} 1-\frac{x}{N-1} &= \frac{N-1}{N-1}-\frac{x}{N-1} \\ &= \frac{N-1-x}{N-1}. \end{aligned}$$

The right-hand side of the first equation above is obtained by setting $1=\frac{N-1}{N-1}$. The probability of not coming in contact with any infecteds, if A contacts are made is,

[1] The correct term would be "*infectious* individuals", but "infecteds" is easier to read and write.

accordingly,

$$\left(\frac{N-1-x}{N-1}\right)^A. \tag{2.1}$$

To see this, assume that $A = 3$. Then, the probability to contract infection during each contact would be $\frac{N-1-x}{N-1} \times \frac{N-1-x}{N-1} \times \frac{N-1-x}{N-1}$. Now, A is not necessarily an integer; in that case, expression (2.1), of course, cannot be written as a repeated product of $\frac{N-1-x}{N-1}$. But that was for illustrative purposes, anyway. The complement of the probability in (2.1) is the probability to come across at least one infected if A contacts are made:

$$1-\left(\frac{N-1-x}{N-1}\right)^A. \tag{2.2}$$

Question 2.b

State some of the assumptions that are necessary for expressions (2.1) and (2.2).

If there are J susceptibles, the expected number of susceptibles who have at least one infectious contact and thus will become infected is[2]

$$J\left(1-\left(\frac{N-1-x}{N-1}\right)^A\right). \tag{2.3}$$

To make the "meaning" of the above expression (2.3) explicit and also to present it as basis for the simulation model to be created, the expression can be rewritten and expanded as follows:

$$x(t+1) = J(t)\left(1-\left(\frac{N(t)-1-x(t)}{N(t)-1}\right)^{A(t)} q\right), \tag{2.4}$$

$$J(t+1) = J(t) - x(t+1), \tag{2.5}$$

$$N(t+1) = N(t) - x(t). \tag{2.6}$$

This formulation implies a discrete (everything happens in discrete intervals) iterative model (the results of one step, $N(t+1)$, $J(t+1)$, and $x(t+1)$, are used in the next iteration). The question about what the time steps correspond to will be kept for later.

I will, however, now get back to the question why A should be interpreted as the transmission coefficient. Considering expression (2.4), it is evident that the number of new infections is only a function of the number of susceptibles, $J(t)$, the size of the population, $N(t)$, the number of currently infectious, $x(t)$, as well as the parameter, $A(t)$. The latter "translates" the number of susceptibles, infecteds, and the total population into new infections. A can actually be interpreted as the number or, rather, rate of contacts that would lead to infection if the other side of the contact is infectious.

[2] This expression has a typo in [1]: The denominator should be $N-1$ instead of $N-$.

Question 2.c

Describe expression (2.3) in statistical terms. Admittedly, this is not a very straightforward question; think of J and the expression in parentheses as two different objects (e.g. probability, etc.).

Even though expression (2.3) contains a probability, the probability to become infected, the model being developed here is not a probabilistic (stochastic) model because the result is always the same.[3]

2.4 Simulation model

Based on this model (Eqs. (2.4)–(2.6)) we are now ready to propose a transmission model. The stated assumptions dictate two important features of the algorithm: It is time-discrete and deterministic. The time-discreteness forces events to happen in discrete time intervals, or rather at defined time points, e.g. at $t = 1, t = 2, t = 3$, etc. The deterministic nature implies that, however often we may realize the simulation, it will always result in the same outcome. En'ko conducted a simulation to create the copious results on which his Table 1 is based–as the translator Klaus Dietz points out, the Table in the original publication was considerably more extensive. We do not know if En'ko used some kind of a mechanical calculator or calculated all numbers with "paper and pencil" himself or had an assistant do the task. The implementation of the simulation is not explicitly described.

2.4.1 Start of the simulation

The start of the simulation, i.e. the initial conditions, are given by what has been stated so far. All the variables (N, x, A, and J) will be indexed by time for transparency ($N(t), x(t), A(t)$, and $J(t)$ for $t \in 1, 2, 3, \ldots$). At the very beginning of the simulation ($t = 0$), we can choose some of the initial conditions according to Table 1. Let us choose the initial conditions of scenario 4 (column 4). Then we will have the following starting point:

t	$N(t)$	$x(t)$	$A(t)$	$J(t)$
0	400	1	$0.01 \times 400 = 4$	200
1	...	...	...	...

[3] We will consider stochastic transmission models in Chap. 6.

Question 2.d

Complete the second line of the above table, using Eqs. (2.4)–(2.6) as well as the relationships that were stated for other variables. Compare your result with the corresponding result from Table 1 (only x is given there).

The best way to systematically compare our simulation with the results shown in Table 1 is to implement it in a spreadsheet program. An example implementation can be found in the online material. The numbers calculated that way are similar, but not identical to the results from Table 1. For example, if the numbers of infected, $x(t)$, are rounded (it is unclear whether En'ko rounded or not), starting with the fourth period the numbers differ by one. This is likely due to a calculation error: If period 4 is set to 15 (instead of 14, rounded from 13.72) then the numbers up to period 10 agree. But these numerical differences are, of course, inconsequential, and we are at a huge advantage in computational power. The comparison merely served to validate our algorithm.

2.4.2 Discussion of Table 1 and Figures

En'ko then discusses Table 1, exploring how the initial number of susceptibles, J, and the transmission parameter A affect the course of the epidemic. He writes:

> *"[I]f by chance or as a consequence of the applied measures the disease disappears for some years, then the number of susceptibles reaches up to one-half of the total population or more; at a new entry of a patient a big epidemic will occur (Nos. 4 and 5), which affects 80–90% of the susceptibles, and the disease (as a consequence of the sanitary-hygienic measures?) will disappear again for some years or will appear in form of rare sporadic cases." (p. 750, first column, fourth paragraph, lines 12–20)*

Question 2.e

What would you answer to En'ko's question embedded in the quotation: "as a consequence of the sanitary-hygienic measures?"

Examination of the scenarios No. 1 trough 39 reveals a few interesting epidemic properties: The following three parameters are varied:

A The number of infectious contacts per individual A/N (generally increases from left to right).

N The size of the "population"; mostly at 400, except for a few exploring lower population numbers.

$J(0)$ Initial number of susceptibles; mostly decreasing from No. 5 through 37.

As a general observation, En'ko states:

> *"For a large quantity A the disease must occur in the form of relatively short, more or less extensive epidemics; under less favourable ratios of the number of*

> *susceptibles with respect to the total size of the population (e.g. in cities, where the children are dispersed between the adults), after an epidemic there will always remain a certain number of susceptibles, who did not become ill; if they are however concentrated, e.g. when the children stay in school, the ratio of the number of susceptibles to the number of insusceptibles remains more favourable for the spread of the disease, and by a new epidemic of a disease, for which a single episode destroys susceptibility, all are affected who did not have the disease earlier[.]" (p. 750, first column, fourth paragraph, line 20 to second column, first paragraph, line 7)*

A few of the statements in this paragraph are particularly interesting. For example, he refers to situations where the level of susceptibility is low, some will always remain susceptible after the epidemic. This is an important observation, and we will acquire the knowledge to understand this in the following chapters. The same "unfavorable condition" can be achieved if the contact rate A is low. If conditions, however, are favorable, all susceptibles will become infected. These properties can be explored with the spreadsheet by modifying the number of susceptible and A.

A little further down, En'ko then observes that, when the contact rate is high and an epidemic

> *"[...] occurs in a very large population, e.g. in a town with a million inhabitants, it must become an endemic."*

Question 2.f

Do you see any evidence of that in the spreadsheet or implicit in anything we have seen so far?

En'ko then proceeds to lead over to the empirical evidence for his model. He comments that, despite the many assumptions that have to be made and the fact that his method is rather crude ("imperfect")

> *"[...] that the observations cannot produce data which can to some extent support the theoretical deductions, but on the contrary, among them there are* exact *data which provide the most splendid support of the theory." (p. 750, second column, second paragraph)*

The observations he is referring to consist, as mentioned before, of infirmary records on measles outbreaks in the period between 1875 and 1888 in a boarding school for girls, the *Imperial Educational College for the Daughters of the Nobility* and the *Alexander Institution* in St Petersburg, Russia. The observations are summarized in the Figure (Fig. 1) and were obtained in two ways:

- The days are recorded when the typical rash appeared.
- The days of transfer of ill children to the infirmary are recorded.

The caption explains which method was used for which epidemic. En'ko then explains the typical course of a measles outbreak:

1. After the first case, 8 to 9 days pass until the next case or cases appear.

2. The number of daily cases then increases until the 12th day and then drops until the 18th day.
3. This behavior defines "quite regular 12-day periods" (p. 750, second column, last paragraph).

This behavior can be seen well in the summary graph (panel j), which combines all outbreaks. He comments on the decreasing amplitude and flattening shape:

> *"[...] the first wave is altogether sharper, the following ones are more flat and the intervals between the maxima are larger." (p. 750, second column, last paragraph)*

He then goes on to explain the first phenomenon, the increasing "smudging" of the peaks:

> *" [...] this depends on the non-simultaneity of the infections and on the variance in the length of the incubation period." (p. 754, first column, first paragraph)*

The second phenomenon, the lengthening of the intervals, is attributed to an interesting mechanism:

> *"[...] by a longer duration of the incubation period of the less susceptibles, who mainly fall sick at the end of the epidemic." (p. 754, first column, first paragraph)*

This explanation alludes to heterogeneity in susceptibility and asserts that those less susceptible would become sick at the end of the epidemic.

Question 2.g

Develop a formal argument of why those less susceptible would become infected later on average.

2.4.3 An important detail: The period

En'ko then introduces the 12-day period of measles. These periods become particularly clear when the data of the cumulative figure (panel j) is divided into 12-day periods and the resulting data added, such that days 1, 13, 25, etc. are added as are days 2, 14, 26, and so on. The result is the table at the top of p. 754, first column:

Day:	1	2	3	4	5	6	7	8	9	10	11	12
Numbers infected:	88	55	43	20	25	11	3	12	29	43	60	74

En'ko explains the 12-day rhythm with the fact that the incubation period (the time from infection to symptom appearance) is about 13 to 14 days, but that, on average, measle infected students infect their peers one or two days before the onset of the rash. The 12-day period is certainly well supported by the data.

This discussion clarifies what this period actually represents: The "usual" time a primary case takes, from the time she was infected, to infect the secondary cases that arise from it. Today, we would call that period "generation time".

Table 2 (p. 752) then tabulates the different epidemics, by period (bottom left, Table 2): 1. period 9–18 days; 2. period 19–30 days, etc. The first period starts at day 9 because

> *"After the first cases of measles there are usually 8–9 days free of measles [...]"* *(p. 750, second column, beginning of last paragraph),*

but may lack a clear biological justification. The epidemics, by period, are shown in the table with the synthetic epidemics that most closely correspond to them. A discussion of the difference between epidemics in the two schools follows which is easy to follow. Then, (second paragraph, second column on p. 754) En'ko compares scarlet fever with measles, mostly with respect to transmissibility. He explains the low transmissibility of scarlet fever, compared to measles, with the fact that the former leads to a sudden onset of the illness and that, therefore, most infected are admitted to the infirmary very early and therefore do not have many opportunities to infect others.

Question 2.h

Is this explanation of transmissibility sufficient?

The paper concludes with the following observation:

> *"The infection of the susceptibles, the dying out of the less resistant, the resulting inheritance of a greater resistance reduce the number of cases and their fatality even without sanitary measures, not excluding vaccination."* *(p. 755, second column, last sentence)*

This offers an interesting evolutionary perspective on the subjects, likely a reflection of Charles Darwin's legacy. However, while evidence of viral evolution is abundant and well accepted, selection for human adaptation to infectious diseases is more elusive.

Appendix 2.A Answers

2.a The population consists of N individuals. Therefore, there are $N-1$ rather than N possible contacts for each individual of that population.

2.b Probabilities (2.1) and (2.2) suggest a discrete time model: while a given individual comes in contact with other members of the population, the number of infecteds remains constant. Presumably, an infectious contact would, possibly with a delay (latent period), result in an increase of the number of infecteds. If this were a continuous time model, more complicated expressions would result. The contacts would have to be indexed by time to relate them to the relevant numbers of infecteds.

2.c J is an integer number–the number of susceptibles–and $\left(1-\left(\frac{N-1-x}{N-1}\right)^{A}\right)$ is the probability of becoming infected (at least one infectious contact) for each of the

J susceptibles. This can therefore be interpreted as a binomial trial, and the numbers infected, x, a binomial random variable such that

$$\Pr(x \mid J, p) = \binom{J}{x} p^x (1-p)^{J-x}$$

where $p = \left(1 - \left(\frac{N-1-x}{N-1}\right)^A\right)$. This is the binomial distribution. The product $Jp = J\left(1 - \left(\frac{N-1-x}{N-1}\right)^A\right)$ is the expected number of infections, $E(x)$, or the mean number of infected.

2.d The values of $N(0)$, $x(0)$, $A(0)$, and $J(0)$ allow us to calculate $x(1)$, the number of infecteds who will infect others in the next iteration of the simulation. Applying formula (2.4), we get

$$\begin{aligned} x(1) &= J(0)\left(1 - \left(\frac{N(0) - 1 - x(0)}{N(0) - 1}\right)^A (0)\right) \\ &= 200 \times \left(1 - \left(\frac{398}{399}\right)^4\right) \\ &= 1.9974. \end{aligned}$$

We then have to calculate the other variables:

$N(1)$ All those who were infectious during the last period are "removed" from the population (sequestered in infirmary); therefore, $N(1) = N(0) - x(0) = 400 - 1 = 399$.

$J(1)$ Similarly, those who became infectious during the current period, $x(1) = 2$, are no longer susceptible, thus $J(1) = J(0) - 2 = 198$.

$A(1)$ A decreases "[...] proportionally to the decline of the population" (p. 750, first column, third paragraph). Therefore $A(1) = A(0) \times \frac{N(1)}{N(0)} = 4 \times \frac{399}{400} = 3.99$.

2.e The answer should be a resounding "No"! The simulated epidemics, such as No. 4&5 affect a majority of the susceptibles: they first increase, then decrease, and finally fully stop. But no "sanitary-hygienic measures" are needed for that! If you are in doubt, study our algorithm to convince yourself that no such element is in the simulation; or look at the spreadsheet (online material).

2.f The conclusion that in a large population the hypothetical illness becomes endemic actually is, in reality, often true. In the context of our observation, however, the conclusion is wrong, especially if infection leads to permanent immunity. The infection could only become endemic if the pool of susceptibles is constantly replenished, either by reproduction or immigration. In our framework, however, we are dealing with *closed* populations. This is even *de facto* the case for quickly developing epidemics that are too rapid for the demographic changes to be of any substantial effect.

2.g Assume that potentially infectious contacts occur between infectious and susceptible individuals at a rate λ and that infection "takes over" a given individual, say individual i, with probability ρ_i. The rate at which a susceptible individual, exactly like i, is infected by one infectious individual is actually $\lambda \times \rho_i$ (the rate λ is diminished by the probability ρ_i). The time to infection of individual i is distributed according to the exponential distribution

$$t \sim \lambda\rho_i \exp(-\lambda\rho_i t).$$

If we pick a particular time, say τ_1, the probability of subject i to still be uninfected (assuming that one infected is on the loose) is given by

$$\Pr(t > \tau_1) = \exp(-\lambda\rho_i\tau_1). \tag{2.7}$$

This is the cumulative distribution function of the exponential distribution. Now let us turn our attention to individual j which has a lower probability, ρ_j, to become infected upon "potentially infectious" contact, i.e. $\rho_j < \rho_i$. At time τ_1 the probability of individual to still be uninfected will be, equivalently to Eq. (2.7),

$$\Pr(t > \tau_1) = \exp(-\lambda\rho_j\tau_1). \tag{2.8}$$

As $\rho_j < \rho_i$ (because the susceptibility of subject j is lower than the one of subject i) the left-hand side of Eq. (2.8) (the probability to survive to time τ_1 uninfected) will be larger than in Eq. (2.7). This means that, at any point in time, more type j individuals will still be susceptible than of type i. This was a somewhat long-winded and indirect argument.

The question can be answered directly as follows. The average time of infection for individuals i is $E(t|i) = \frac{1}{\rho_i\tau_1}$, and for individuals j it is $E(t|j) = \frac{1}{\rho_j\tau_1}$; this is simply a property of the exponential distribution. As ρ_j is smaller than ρ_i, the opposite must be true for the respective fractions. Therefore, the average time to infection is later for the less than the more susceptible individuals.

2.h This explanation of transmissibility which is purely based on disease-specific opportunities for transmission is not sufficient to fully explain differences in transmissibility. Even though opportunity to transmit is important, biological properties of the infectious agent are extremely important, too. Such properties include, e.g. in the case of viral diseases, the affinity of the virus to (in our case) human cells, its ability to efficiently reproduce in human cells and to be excreted by its human host. As an aside: The bacterial etiology of scarlet fever was already known at En'ko's time, but it is unclear whether he was specifically aware of that. The concept of a viral etiology became not into life until the early 20th century.

Appendix 2.B Supplementary material

Supplementary material related to this chapter can be found online at http://dx.doi.org/10.1016/B978-0-12-802260-3.00002-X.

References

[1] P.D. En'ko, On the course of epidemics of some infectious diseases, International Journal of Epidemiology 18 (4) (1989) 749–755.

W.H. Hamer (1906) and H. Soper (1929): Why diseases come and go

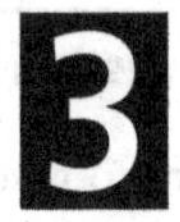

Contents

3.1 Introduction

This chapter discusses two companion papers that were separated by more than two decades and connected by an asymmetric relationship: Soper's later paper [1] somewhat deferentially refers to and acknowledges Hamer's earlier contribution [2]. Following the sequence of these two papers, I will first discuss Hamer's paper and then Soper's.

3.2 Hamer: Variability and persistence

3.2.1 A tortuous introduction

Hamer read his paper in 1906 before the Royal College of Physicians of London as Milroy Lecture: The introductory paragraphs, spanning from page 733 to the top of page 734, start with a mention of influenza epidemics during the 19th century, transitions to epidemics of "throat distemper". Especially for "throat distemper" and continued fevers, Hamer recognizes a great difficulty in identifying "persistency of type". From a modern perspective, these passages seem somewhat obscure, and their goal is not immediately obvious.

A Historical Introduction to Mathematical Modeling of Infectious Diseases. DOI: 10.1016/B978-0-12-802260-3.00003-1

Question 3.a

Try to give an interpretation of the introductory paragraphs: What is their purpose?

After discussing the case of tuberculosis which had been declining in mortality over decades, Hamer finally turns his attention to the real focal point of the lecture by stating:

> *"It is generally admitted that the persistency of type displayed by* measles *and* small-pox *is quite remarkable. For that reason they afford specially promising material for study of short period waves, and in turning therefore to the examination of variability of type these two diseases may with advantage be considered in the first instance. The simplest case is that of the short period waves of measles." (p. 734, first column, second paragraph)*

3.2.2 Characteristic of periodic measles epidemics

Hamer comments on the, on average, biennial periodicity of measles[1] epidemic, quoting Arthur Whitelegge who published several papers on epidemic disease in the late 19th century (no specific source given):

> *"[Explosions in towns occur commonly at about biennial intervals] when the accumulation of susceptible persons is sufficient and the climatic and other internal conditions offer sufficiently small resistance." (p. 734, first column, beginning of second paragraph)*

This clearly demonstrates that the idea of the crucial role "accumulation of susceptibles" in the periodicity of infectious disease incidence was ripe by the time of Hamer's lecture. Hamer then importantly notes:

> *"The problem (in the case of measles in a large community) is simplified for the reasons that we are dealing with an obligatory parasite. [...] Furthermore, one attack confers almost complete protection." (p. 734, first column, second paragraph)*

Question 3.b

Why is the being an "obligatory parasite" and full immunity after infection important in this context? Note that there is no single right answer.

In the following paragraphs, the following important assumptions about measle epidemiology in London, on which the following derivations will be based, are identified (page 734, first column, third paragraph, as well as following paragraphs set in small print):

[1] At the time of Hamer's lecture, the viral nature of the agent of measles was unknown. Viruses had actually only recently been differentiated from bacteria as "filterable agents" that passed through a ceramic filter.

- Case fatality of measles is 1.5%.
- Maximum weekly number of measles cases: 6,400 (160 deaths), declining after an interval of 39 weeks to a minimum of 400 (10 deaths). These numbers were obtained by "first plotting out weekly figures for periods selected as presenting typical epidemic movement and then superimposing one wave upon another [...]".
- This results in an epidemic period of approx. 18 months with maxima occurring alternatively in summers and winters.
- The population of London is augmented by 2,500 susceptible people, mostly infants; taking into consideration mortality, as well as the "comparative insusceptibility of very young infants" (see Question 3.c) he settles at a weekly rate of increase, or 2,200.
- The incubation period of measles is two weeks.

Question 3.c

Hamer states that to the population of London, each week, approximately by "[...] 2,500 susceptibles, or, allowing for the comparative insusceptibility of young infants [...], say by 2,200 susceptibles". What modern interpretation of "comparative insusceptibility of young infants" could immunological considerations offer?

Referring to the only figure of the article, Hamer then infers important epidemiologic features of measles in London, based on the stated assumptions and estimates epidemiologic quantities. The x-axis of the graph (M to N) is the time axis, and y-axis represents a rate. For the epidemic curve this would be the measles incidence rate, for the horizontal line (D to E) the rate at which susceptibles are added, which is constant. Up to the point labeled A which represents a local maximum of the epidemic curve and the first value displayed, the number of cases is increasing. The number of cases is then decreasing until K, the (local) nadir of the synthetic epidemic curve displayed in the figure. The points B and C represent "inflection points": He then importantly states:

> *"In passing these points increase is converted into decrease, or vice versa, the tangent to the curve at the instant being horizontal and stationary. It will be apparent, therefore, that at A each case may be regarded as infecting one other case; this will also hold good at K." (p. 734, first column, fourth paragraph, set in small font)*

Note that these inflection points are defined by the intersection of the epidemic curve (number of cases by unit of time (= incidence rate)) and the horizontal line that represents the steady rate at which new susceptibles are added to the population: This intersection corresponds to the moment in time:

> *"If the virulence of the measles organism and other factors be assumed to be the same at A and K, it will follow, inasmuch as each case is then capable of infecting one other case, that the* ***number of susceptible persons in the population at those points of time will be identical****." (boldface not in original; p. 734, first column, fourth paragraph, set in small font)*

The realization that the number of susceptibles will be the same at such opposite stages of the epidemic is arguably the most important of Hamer's achievements in his lecture.

Question 3.d

Consider the statement in the previous quotation: "[...] each case may be regarded as infecting one other case." Comment on what that may mean for an epidemic curve. Derive the fact that the numbers of susceptibles at point A (peak) and point K (nadir) are, in the discussed synthetic epidemic, identical.

Hamer then proceeds to derive the number of susceptibles at the signature points of the curve: at maximum, A, at the first inflection point, B, at the minimum, K, and the second inflection point, C. His derivation is based on the equality of the areas ADB and BHK and the following approximation: The area ABD will be larger than

$$\frac{AD \times DB}{2} = \frac{(6{,}400 - 2{,}200) \times 14}{2} \approx 30{,}000,$$

because this corresponds to the triangle defined by the points A, D, and B. The distance AD is calculated as the maximum "excess case rate", i.e. the maximal incidence rate (6,400 cases per week) minus the rate at which susceptibles are added (2,200 per week). The distance DB is the amount of time (in weeks) from the peak to the first "inflection point", i.e. 14 weeks (top second column, page 734). The area of that triangle is, as implied by Hamer, smaller than the area ABD. This can be mathematically proven, but even more easily can be contemplating the "overhang" to the right between the line AB and the curve.

Question 3.e

Try to show why, given the assumptions presented, the areas ABD and BHK are identical.

To calculate the absolute (as opposed to relative) numbers of susceptibles at the time points that correspond to A, B, K, C, and Z, Hamer argues as follows: In the "neighborhood" of B the number of cases fall from 2,500 to 2,000 in the room of 14 days. The implication here is that 2,500 cases infected with measles give rise to 2,000 cases because the "incubation period" of measles is about that period of time. By "incubation period" Hamer is likely referring to the generation time (therefore the "quotes"). Implicitly, Hamer treats the system, at least partly, in a discrete fashion: The cases in week k will be responsible for all the cases in week $k+1$ and for none beyond. Around B the number of susceptibles must be such that one case infects $\frac{2{,}000}{2{,}500} = \frac{4}{5}$–therefore, the number of susceptibles at B must be $\frac{4}{5}$ of the susceptibles at A, which we denote by x. Hamer expresses this in the following equation:

$$\frac{x - 30{,}000}{x} = \frac{4}{5}. \tag{3.1}$$

This equation can be easily solved for x as will be demonstrated. Solving a simple equation in one unknown is basic algebra; for readers with "rusty" mathematical skills this is demonstrated here:

$$\begin{aligned}
\frac{x-30{,}000}{x} &= \frac{4}{5},\\
\text{(Multiply both sides by } x\text{)}\ x-30{,}000 &= \frac{4}{5}\times x,\\
\text{(Add 30,000 to both sides)}\ x &= \frac{4}{5}x+30{,}000,\\
\text{(Subtract } \tfrac{4}{5}x \text{ from both sides)}\ x-\frac{4}{5}x &= 30{,}000,\\
\text{(Simplify the left-hand side)}\ x\left(1-\frac{4}{5}\right) &= 30{,}000,\\
\text{(Divide both sides by } \left(1-\tfrac{4}{5}\right)\text{)}\ x &= \frac{30{,}000}{1-\frac{4}{5}},\\
\text{(Simplify the right-hand side)}\ x &= \frac{30{,}000}{\frac{4}{5}},\\
x &= 30{,}000\times 5 = 150{,}000.
\end{aligned}$$

The solution to the question of "how many susceptibles x are there at point B?" therefore is $x = 150{,}00$.

> **Note**
>
> The logical analysis of Fig. 7 is, in my view, the greatest of Hamer's achievements in this paper. Hamer's ingenuity necessary to construct the, somewhat counterintuitive, trajectory of susceptibles, given the incidence curve and a set of basic assumptions, has to be emphasized.

Given the knowledge of x, i.e. of the number of susceptibles at A (150,000), the numbers of susceptibles can then be calculated for the points B (120,000), K (150,000: has to be equal to the number at A–see above), C (180,000) and Z (150,000: has to be equal to the number at A and K). Hamer then writes:

> *"A C the condition* $\frac{x+30}{x} = \frac{2{,}000}{2{,}500}$, *if applied, would give a somewhat lower value of x that the one already obtained. In other words, the curve cannot be exactly symmetrical in relation to ordinates drawn through H K L, and if we wish to be precise it should be 'skewed' accordingly." (p. 734, second column, first paragraph, set in small font)*

> **Question 3.f**
>
> Can you spot an inconsistency in this quoted passage, particularly in the equation?

3.2.3 The case of influenza

Hamer then turns his attention to influenza, the epidemiology of which he tries to explain from the insights gained by the examination of measles. He then writes:

> *"Assume each case of influenza, at the commencement of an epidemic capable of infecting, say, two fresh cases, and take the incubation periods one third of a week, then in first week one, two, and four cases; in the second week eight, 16, and 32, will be attacked, and so on. As, however, larger numbers of those specially exposed (city men, theater-goers, etc.) are stricken down the rate of increase will necessarily slacken." (p. 734, second column, end of third paragraph, set in small font)*

Question 3.g

Discuss, in the context of his reasoning for measles, Hamer's explanation of the epidemiologic dynamics of influenza.

3.3 Soper: Periodicity in disease prevalence

Soper read his paper "before the Royal Statistical Society" in 1929, over two decades after Hamer gave his lecture. He modestly acknowledges, at the end of the introductory paragraph, that

> *"In this research I was merely following up the trail blazed by Sir William Hamer more than twenty years ago, only in detail departing from his method." (p. 35, second paragraph)*

He then begins his formal treatment of the periodicity of measles epidemics by defining fundamental concepts.

"Regeneration" of the population

Susceptibles are drafted into the population, by either birth or immigration, at the rate a such that in the infinitesimal time interval dt an "amount"[2] $a \times dt$ $(= adt)$ susceptibles are added to the population. These added susceptibles are characterized by three features: First, equal susceptibility to infectious agent under study; second, equal ability to transmit; and, third, once no longer transmitting, the "individual" will "pass out" of observation.[3]

"Law of infection"

Soper then discusses several models of transmissibility over time to settle on one according to which all infective power is concentrated at the end of a constant interval.

[2] Note that this treatment of the epidemic process does not treat a population as made up of certain numbers of susceptible, infectious, etc. individuals, but, rather, of "quantities" of these types.

[3] Hence, that state is, in the modeling literature, commonly referred to as "removed" or R-state.

He assumes that the "instantaneous power of infection" occurs at the end of the incubation period.[4] Referring to Fig. 2 he postulates that, when approaching the condition of "instantaneous power of infection", the number of new infections in the interval (A, B) depends on the number of new infections in the interval $(A, B) - t$, where t is the incubation period.

Mass action

The transmission process is driven by "mass action", a concept developed in the mid-19th century chemistry: Without further delving into a discussing of the chemical theory,[5] it suffices to emphasize the meaning of this analogy: *Mass action* implies that the rate of a chemical reaction is proportional of the amount or concentration of reagents present. Applied to the transmission process, this is obvious, given the assumption that the number of secondary cases generated by one case is proportional to the number (proportion of) susceptibles in the population "at this instant".

Question 3.h

What *instant* is Soper referring to?

Therefore, if the number of susceptibles determines, "other things equal", how many secondary cases result from a case, there must be an equilibrium number of susceptibles, when one case infects another (and *only* one). Soper denotes this number by m and argues (fifth paragraph, p. 37) that if there are x susceptibles, each case will result in $\frac{x}{m}$ cases. This assertion is a direct consequence of the "mass action" and in tradition of Hamer's thinking. However, no stringent justification is given, neither by Hamer nor Soper.

Question 3.i

Why, given the stated assumptions, does one case give rise to $\frac{x}{m}$ (secondary) cases?

To make "the synthetic epidemics to [...] not depend on the absolute sizes of communities" Soper introduces the "time element" s such that

$$m = s\,a.$$

This equation can be interpreted as follows: As a is the rate at which susceptibles are recruited (number of susceptible per time), when multiplied by a given length of time (s) a number of susceptibles (m) results. As we have seen, that number m is the "equilibrium number" of susceptibles ("one gives one"). Given a, the time parameter s

[4] The incubation period refers to the time period after becoming infected that is symptom-free. Illness onset is after the end of the incubation period. The period from the time of infection to the time when infectiousness starts is widely referred to as *latent period* (see any textbook of infectious disease epidemiology). The assumption that infectiousness is concentrated at the end of the incubation period implies that latent period and incubation period are (practically) identical.

[5] I would not be capable of doing so.

therefore characterizes a population: a large s (long time to accumulate m susceptibles) implies that there are "few interminglings of the sort that conduce to infection".

3.3.1 Infection dynamics

From what was discussed so far and assuming that "$z\,dt$ are the cases"[6] and that the unit of time is the "incubation" period[7] τ, the basic equation for the infection dynamic should not come as a surprise:

$$z = \frac{x}{m} \times z_{-1}$$

where the suffix represents a time index. Because "the change in x [...] is usually small in the unit interval (about a fortnight for measles)" Soper proposes the following notation:

$$\frac{z_{\frac{1}{2}}}{z_{-\frac{1}{2}}} = \frac{x}{m} = \frac{x}{s\,a} \tag{3.2}$$

or

$$\frac{\text{no. of cases next interval}}{\text{no. of cases last interval}} = \frac{\text{no. of susceptibles at present interval}}{s \times \text{accessions per interval}}.$$

Question 3.j

Explain the denominator, $s\,a$ in the right-most expression of Eq. (3.2).

To be entirely consistent, the equation should be written as

$$\frac{z_t}{z_{t-1}} = \frac{x_t}{m}$$

where t represents the current time. In this interpretation, x_t would represent the relevant level of susceptibility: Exactly at the moment, when all those that became infected at time $t-1$ dispose of all their infectivity (at time t). Note that this is the framework for a time-discrete system, when everything happens in steps at times t, $t+1$, $t+2$, etc.

3.3.2 The simulated epidemic

Fig. 3 represents a "synthetic" epidemic based on machine calculations[8] based on Eq. (3.2) and supposing that

[6] This implies that z is the rate at which cases are generated; note that dt is the "infinitesimal time" element.
[7] In modern terminology, *latent* period; this term will be used henceforth when Soper refers to "incubation" period.
[8] Given the chronology, such machine must have been a mechanical calculator, widely used at the end of the 19th and beginning of the 20th century.

"[...] 1000 susceptibles added each interval, or step, and taking $s = 20, 30, 40, 50$, so that the steady state numbers of susceptibles are 20,000, 30,000, 40,000 and 50,000. A start was made at a peak, with $z_{-\frac{1}{2}}$ equal to $z_{\frac{1}{2}}$, and consequently $x = m$. The successive values of x are obtained by adding 1,000 susceptibles each time and subtracting the number of cases in the last or preceding interval. [...] A rather serious epidemic starting-point was taken, namely, when the cases were four times the accessions (that is, four times the number of cases characterizing a steady state, without oscillations) [...]."

Question 3.k

With $s = 40$ and $m = 40{,}000$ and using the described starting point, implement this epidemic (using MS Excel, R or any other software platform).

3.3.3 Periods

Soper states that, "if the incubation interval is τ, the equation of the epidemic curve of the kind presupposed is":

$$\frac{z_{\frac{1}{2}}\tau}{z_{-\frac{1}{2}}\tau} = \frac{x}{m} \tag{3.3}$$

where z denotes the "cases per unit time"; z therefore is a rate–in epidemiological terms, this might be called *incidence rate*.

Note

The notation of this expression is not entirely clear: Is τ supposed to be in the subscript of z such that it reads $z_{\frac{1}{2}\tau}$, the incidence rate half an "incubation" (latent) interval removed from the present instant? Or should it read $z_{\frac{1}{2}}\tau$ as the text suggests? In that case, the meaning would be: The incidence rate half a time interval from the present multiplied by the "incubation" period. I suggest that the intended notation for expression (3.3) should be

$$\frac{z_{\frac{1}{2}\tau}}{z_{-\frac{1}{2}\tau}} = \frac{x}{m}. \tag{3.4}$$

Fundamentally, expression (3.3), or rather (3.4), appears to imply once more a discrete-time system: Everything, i.e. the recruitment of susceptibles and their transformation into "cases" that are, in turn, able to produce more cases, happens at discrete time steps. Eq. (3.3) would be more consistent with that framework in the form

$$\frac{z_t}{z_{t-1}} = \frac{x_t}{m}.$$

The ratio between the number of cases in the current interval to the number of cases in the previous interval (which produced them) is *only* a function of the number of susceptibles in the current interval compared to the number of "steady state" number of susceptibles. That ratio can be interpreted as *effective reproduction number*, an extremely important concept in transmission modeling that we will encounter again. Furthermore,

$$\frac{dx}{dt} = a - z \tag{3.5}$$

which translates to: The rate of change in the number of susceptibles (x) over time (left-hand side) equals the difference between the rate at which susceptibles are added (a) and the rate at which susceptibles are removed (z); if the rate at which cases are produced (z, which is variable) is larger than the rate at which susceptibles are produced (a, which is constant) the "net change" in susceptibles ($\frac{dx}{dt}$) will be negative (i.e. loss of susceptibles) and *vice versa*. If both sides of Eq. (3.5) are integrated with respect to time from t_0 to t_1 and the time $t_0 = 0$ when the number of susceptibles is at the equilibrium level m, the following expression for the number of susceptibles as a function of time is obtained:

$$\begin{aligned}
\frac{dx(t)}{dt} &= a - z(t), \\
\int_0^{t_1} \frac{dx(t)}{dt} dt &= \int_0^{t_1} a - z(t) dt \text{ (integrate both sides)}, \\
\int_0^{t_1} dx(t) &= \int_0^{t_1} (a - z(t))\, dt \\
& \quad \text{(}dt \text{ cancels from left-hand side; separating } a \text{ and } z\text{)}, \\
x(t)\big|_0^{t_1} &= \int_0^{t_1} (a - z(t))\, dt \; \Big(\int dx(t) = x(t) + C; \\
& \quad \text{the } C \text{ falls away calculating definite integral)}, \\
x(t) - m &= \int_0^{t_1} (a - z(t))\, dt \text{ (left-hand side: } x(0) = m\text{)}, \\
x(t) &= m + \int_0^{t_1} (a - z(t))\, dt \text{ (add } m \text{ to both sides).}
\end{aligned} \tag{3.6}$$

Derivation of the period

Let $z = a \exp(u)$, where u is, according to Soper, an "index measure of cases." This expression may seem somewhat cryptic, but it is crucial for the following derivation. Let us therefore try to shed light on its meaning. The literal "translation" of the expression equates the case incidence at a given time to the constant rate at which susceptibles are "created", a, multiplied by the exponent of a number, u, which depends on the number of cases present, but also on the number of susceptibles. We actually know exactly how many new cases are created in a given interval (z_t): This would be the number of cases in the preceding interval, z_{t-1}, multiplied by the ratio, we know so well by now, $\frac{x_t}{m}$.

Question 3.I

Find an expression for u.

This translates to

$$z_t = z_{t-1} \frac{x_t}{m}. \tag{3.7}$$

We have seen before that the "equilibrium" number of susceptibles (when one case gives rise to one) m can be expressed as $m = s\,a$. We can therefore write Eq. (3.7) as

$$z_t = z_{t-1} \frac{x_t}{s\,a}. \tag{3.8}$$

Using the equality $z_t = a \exp(u_t)$ in (3.4), we get:

$$\begin{aligned} \frac{\exp(u_{\frac{1}{2}\tau})}{\exp(u_{-\frac{1}{2}\tau})} &= \exp(u_{\frac{1}{2}\tau} - u_{-\frac{1}{2}\tau}) \text{ (basic properties of exponents)} \\ &= \exp(\delta_\tau u) \\ &= \frac{x}{m}. \end{aligned} \tag{3.9}$$

The substitution $u_{\frac{1}{2}\tau} - u_{-\frac{1}{2}\tau}$ with $\delta_\tau u$, according to Soper "in the usual notation", has the following meaning: the difference in u between $-\frac{1}{2}\tau$ before and $\frac{1}{2}\tau$ after the present instant. If the changes in u are "small" in that interval, i.e. if $\delta_\tau u$ is "small" then $\exp(\delta_\tau u) = 1 + \delta_\tau u$.

The approximation $\lim_{x \to 0} \exp(x) = 1 + x$ is often useful.[a] This somewhat mystical expression can, however, be understood from the series representation of $\exp(x)$, i.e.

$$\exp(x) = \sum_{k=0}^{\infty} \frac{x^k}{k!}$$

where $k! = \prod_{j=1}^{k} j = k \times (k-1) \times (k-2) \times \cdots \times 1$ ("k factorial"). Note that $0! = 1$ and that the explicit product $k \times (k-1) \times \cdots$ shown above is only possible for $k \geq 4$. If x is small, say 0.01, then the series becomes

$$\begin{aligned} \exp(0.01) &= \frac{0.01^0}{0!} + \frac{0.01^1}{1!} + \frac{0.01^2}{2!} + \frac{0.01^3}{3!} + \cdots \\ &= \frac{1}{1} + \frac{0.01}{1} + \frac{0.0001}{2} + \frac{0.000001}{6} + \cdots \\ &= 1 + 0.01 + 0.00005 + 1.666667E - 07 + \cdots \\ &\approx 1 + 0.01 \end{aligned}$$

because the terms after the second term become negligible.

[a] This notation expresses an equality when x approaches 0.

Question 3.m

Is u likely "small"? Use your expression for u and your "synthetic epidemic".

Thus, Soper states that

$$\exp(\delta_\tau u) = 1 + \delta_\tau u \tag{3.10}$$
$$= 1 + \tau \frac{du}{dt}. \tag{3.11}$$

The =-sign in (3.10) above should actually be replaced by an ≈-sign because it is an approximate relationship. The latter equality provided by Soper may require some explanation.[9] He writes

$$\delta_\tau u = \tau \frac{du}{dt}. \tag{3.12}$$

To remind us, $\delta_\tau u$ is the change in u over the period τ. The right-hand side of the expression, $\tau \frac{du}{dt}$, represents the "instantaneous change" in u or the rate of change multiplied by the incubation period τ. If the rate of change is constant in the interval then this equality holds true. A notational problem with this expression, however, that appears to be a theme here, is the lack of a time index associated with u. A less ambiguous way to express it would be $\tau \frac{du(t)}{dt}$ because otherwise it is unclear what "instantaneous change" it is referring to. Furthermore, I believe $\delta_\tau u$ is intended to read $\delta(t)_u$: Otherwise the expression would suggest that δ_τ is multiplied by u, which is not the case. Once we have accepted the equality (3.12), we can write

$$1 + \tau \frac{du}{dt} = \frac{x}{m}.$$

This equality holds because of (3.10) and (3.9). Once this is established, both sides of expression (3.12) can be differentiated:

$$\tau \frac{du(t)}{dt} = \frac{x(t)}{m},$$
$$\tau \frac{d^2u(t)}{dt^2} = \frac{1}{m}\frac{dx(t)}{dt} \text{ (taking derivative of both sides)},$$
$$\tau \frac{d^2u(t)}{dt^2} = \frac{a - z(t)}{m} \text{ (taking derivative of both sides)},$$
$$\tau \frac{d^2u(t)}{dt^2} = \frac{a - a\exp(u(t))}{m} \text{ (substituting for } z(t)),$$
$$\tau \frac{d^2u(t)}{dt^2} = \frac{a(1 - \exp(u(t)))}{m} \text{ (factoring out } a), \tag{3.13}$$
$$\tau \frac{d^2u(t)}{dt^2} = \frac{(1 - \exp(u(t)))}{s} \text{ (replacing } \frac{a}{m} \text{ with } \frac{1}{s}), \tag{3.14}$$

[9] Especially for those among us whose calculus skills are somewhat shaky.

$$\frac{d^2u(t)}{dt^2} = \frac{(1-\exp(u(t)))}{s\tau} \text{ (dividing both sides by } \tau\text{)}, \tag{3.15}$$

$$\frac{d^2u(t)}{dt^2} \approx \frac{1-1-u(t)}{s\tau}$$

$$\text{(replacing } \exp(u(t)) \text{ with the approximation } 1+u(t)\text{)}, \tag{3.16}$$

$$\frac{d^2u(t)}{dt^2} \approx \frac{-u(t)}{s\tau}. \tag{3.17}$$

Soper presents the above expression at the bottom by subtracting the right-hand expression, $\frac{-u(t)}{s\tau}$, from both sides, i.e.

$$\frac{d^2u(t)}{dt^2} + \frac{u(t)}{s\tau} = 0. \tag{3.18}$$

Note that the =-sign should strictly be replaced by the ≈-sign ("approximately is") because of the approximation $\exp(u(t)) \approx 1 + u(t)$. The presentation of (3.18) is followed by the statement:

> *"Thus small epidemics under the conditions assumed are cyclic and period = $2\pi\sqrt{s\tau}$" (p. 40, first sentence)*

where $s = \frac{m}{a}$. This may, for the uninitiated, seem utterly obscure. It can, however, be justified as follows. After subtracting $\frac{u(t)}{s\tau}$ from both sides, Eq. (3.18) becomes

$$\frac{d^2u(t)}{dt^2} = -\frac{1}{s\tau}u(t). \tag{3.19}$$

What this really tells us is this: The second derivative of the function $u(t)$ (left-hand side) is the negative of that function, divided by $s\tau$ (right-hand side). This holds true for the two trigonometric functions sine and cosine:

$$\frac{d^2}{dt^t}(\cos bt) = -b^2 \cos bt. \tag{3.20}$$

The $-b^2$ in front of the cosine on the right-hand side of (3.20) can be understood as a result from applying the chain rule: To take the derivative of the function $\cos g(t)$ with respect to t, the derivative of that function with respect to $g(t)$ is taken, which is $-\sin g(t)$. Then, the derivative of $g(t)$ with respect to t is taken. Here, $g(t) = bt$ and $\frac{d}{dt}bt = b$.

Furthermore,

$$\begin{aligned} \frac{d^2}{dt^2}(\cos bt) &= -b\frac{d}{dt}(\sin bt) \\ &= -b^2 \cos bt. \end{aligned} \tag{3.21}$$

Note that b is a real constant. In analogy to Eq. (3.19), it becomes clear that b^2 corresponds to $s\tau$ and thus $b = \frac{1}{\sqrt{s\tau}}$. The implication of expression (3.21) is that

$$u(t) = \cos\frac{1}{\sqrt{s\tau}}t. \tag{3.22}$$

A quick note on this result is in order. Even though what we derived is not really wrong, we actually should have stated Eq. (3.22) as

$$u(t) = D\cos\frac{1}{\sqrt{s\tau}}t \tag{3.23}$$

where D is a real constant. This is because

$$\frac{d^2}{dt^t}(D\cos bt) = -Db^2\cos bt.$$

The effect of D is *only* on the amplitude, but not on the period of the function; and it could be any D. We therefore cannot make any statements regarding the number of infections, only how frequently epidemics occur.

If the argument of the cosine is measured in radians then $\cos 0 = \cos 2\pi = \cos 4\pi = \cdots$, i.e. the local maximum of the cosine at 0 repeats at 2π, 4π, 6π, etc. In other words, the period is 2π. If the argument of cosine is $v = bt$, the period is simply inflated (or deflated if $b > 1$) by the factor $\frac{1}{b}$.

Returning to expressions (3.19) and (3.21) and setting $b = \frac{1}{\sqrt{s\tau}}$ and $\frac{1}{b} = \sqrt{s\tau}$, it therefore becomes clear that the period of this system must be $2\pi\sqrt{s\tau}$. The "obscure" relationship thus appears justified.

Question 3.n

We now have two "competing" expressions for $u(t)$: the one derived in the answer to Question 3.h; the other one represented in Eq. (3.22). Are the two expressions actually equal? Verify, using $u(t)$, for $t \in \{1, \ldots, 100\}$ ($\in$ reads "in").

If we set $\sqrt{s\tau}$ to be the unit of time, i.e. let $\sqrt{s\tau} = s\tau = 1$ (square root of one is one), Eq. (3.15) becomes

$$\frac{d^2u(t)}{dt^2} = 1 - \exp(u(t)) \quad (\text{as } \frac{1}{\sqrt{s\tau}} = \frac{1}{s\tau} = 1),$$

Eq. (8) in Soper's paper. Similarly, if the "incubation period" τ is chosen as the unit of time, as assumed for the "synthetic epidemic", then it becomes

$$\frac{d^2u(t)}{dt^2} = \frac{1}{s}(1 - \exp(u(t))) \quad (\text{as } \tau = 1 \text{ and thus } \frac{1}{s\tau} = \frac{1}{s}),$$

Eq. (9) in the article and the period, for small oscillations, $2\pi\sqrt{s}$. This formula is used for the following table (p. 40):

	s			
	20	30	40	50
Period $= 2\pi\sqrt{s}$	28.1	34.4	39.7	44.4

For "fourfold epidemics", where at the peak the number of infections per period are four times the addition of susceptibles (a) increase, as Soper writes, the period by around 13% compared to the periods of small oscillations (see "period" tab, online Supplement) and then speculates that the addition of a cases at peak may add 4.5% to the period.[10]

Question 3.o

Is this guess of Soper, that each addition of $a = 1000$ cases to the epidemic peak increases the period, compared to the small oscillation case, by about 3.5%, on target? (Note that you could use the spreadsheet in online Supplement to examine this question.)

In the second paragraph of page 1929, Soper then comments on the trajectories of susceptibles and cases, in particular during the inter-epidemic periods when there are very few cases. Susceptibles linearly increase at the rate of "renewal", a, resulting in a saw-tooth pattern (Fig. 4). Cases, on the other hand, increase from period j to period $j+1$ by the factor $\frac{m+aj}{m}$. Soper remarks on the resulting "inverse of a *poisson*"; I was not able to decipher the meaning of that. The name of the French 19th century mathematician *Siméon Denis Poisson* is today most intimately associated with the Poisson distribution, but this cannot be the intended meaning here. Furthermore, the graph shown in Fig. 5, which is u-shaped (concave), cannot be explained by this pattern of increase (strictly increasing).

3.3.4 Considerations of seasonal factors and model fit to Glasgow data

In the second part of the paper, entitled "§2. The Point Infection Curve modified by Seasonal Change in Infectivity. Analysis of a Glasgow Composite Measles Curve. Synthetic Curves of Epidemic Measles," Soper examines the monthly measles incidence data from Glasgow, Scotland, 1888 to 1927 and makes an effort to fit his transmission model to this data. The following third part, entitled "§3. Analysis of a Sequence of Years. Prediction," may be devoted to an attempt to make the model more "realistic", i.e. more similar to the monthly Glasgow data. Parts two and three are actually considerably more expansive than the first part, but I will focus on the parts and aspects that can profit from some explanations and will not dwell on passages that, I believe, are more easily comprehended or, from a modern perspective, of little relevance. Rather, I will try to outline the ideas and approaches that are innovative and original.

Seasonal dynamics

Soper grants that his simple recursive model (3.2) does not really explain real time series of measles incidence, such as the Glasgow data, very well and contemplates the possibility that transmission may be modified by a seasonal factor. The argument he

[10] We should remind us that Soper did not have access to powerful computation that we have at our fingertips!

develops begins by adopting Soper's assumption of an equilibrium ("level") number of susceptibles ($= M$) being equivalent to 70 weeks' accumulation.[11]

As the mean number of cases of measles over the six two-year periods ("biennia") for the "composite curve", i.e. the six two-year periods added, per week is 1,250 the equilibrium number for Glasgow is $M = a \times s = 1{,}250 \times 70 = 87{,}500$. This number is then used by Soper to reconstruct the monthly numbers of susceptibles, as the susceptibles in one month are the numbers at the beginning of the previous month with the cases in the previous month subtracted.

As the Glasgow data is recorded in monthly intervals (~ 4 weeks), while the "incubation period" (or more appropriately, generation time) is i months (in the case of 2 weeks, i would be 0.5), the per-generation increase in the number of cases would be by the factor $\left(\frac{x_{t+1}}{x_t}\right)^i$, where the index t represents months.

The reason for that can be seen in the following example. Assume that the generation time is half a month, i.e. $i = 0.5$. In the first epidemic generation ($=$ period) there are 10 cases that double to 20, then 40, and finally 80 in the following periods. Clearly the factor of increase is

$$\frac{z_2}{z_1} = \frac{20}{10} = \frac{z_3}{z_2} = \cdots = 2,$$

i.e. the number of cases doubles with each generation. If we consider months now, we will have $10 + 20 = 30$ in the first month and $40 + 80 = 120$ in the second month. The month-to-month increase factor will therefore be $\frac{120}{30} = 4$. If we raise this number to the power of $i = 0.4$, we get $4^0 \cdot 5 = 2$, i.e. we have recovered the doubling factor calculated first. This, however, only works if the rate of increase is constant over the month.

Based on these considerations, Soper formulates Eq. (11) on p. 42:

$$\left(\frac{z_{\frac{1}{2}}}{z_{-\frac{1}{2}}}\right)^i = k_\theta \frac{x}{m} \tag{3.24}$$

where k_θ is the seasonal transmission factor, θ representing a particular month. This factor can either increase ($k_\theta < 1$) or increase $k_\theta > 1$ the influence of the current number of susceptible on the number of cases resulting from the current cases. To be consistent with the notation I proposed before, Eq. (3.24) should be written as

$$\left(\frac{z_t}{z_{t-1}}\right)^i = k_{\theta_t} \frac{x_t}{m}. \tag{3.25}$$

Taking the natural logarithm of both sides, we get

$$i \log(z_t) - \log(z_{t-1}) \quad = \quad i\delta \log(z_t),$$

[11] I have not found Hamer's specific reference to these 70 weeks; however, he states that the equilibrium number of susceptibles for London is 150,000 ($= M$); assuming a weekly influx of 2,200 susceptibles (a) it would take 68 weeks (s) to accumulate M susceptibles. Soper likely just rounded that number to 70.

$$i\delta \log(z_t) \quad = \quad \log(k_{\theta_t}) + \log(x_t) - \log(m). \tag{3.26}$$

Note that the logarithmic transformation leads to addition/subtraction rather than multiplication/division, and to multiplication instead of power (in the case of i). Also, $i\log(z_t) - \log(z_{t-1})$ is "renamed" to $i\delta\log(z_t)$.

The process by which Soper comes up with the seasonal factor k_θ (I have been writing it as k_{θ_t}) is not described with much detail, and I will simply outline it here. He basically examines the error of the simple model (number of new cases only as a function of previous cases and ratio of susceptibles to equilibrium number of susceptibles) when contrasted with the composite curve which adds the six biennial periods, such that the number of the first "month" (four week interval) of the 1901/2 period is added to the corresponding number of the 1903/4, 1905/6, etc. periods. The monthly– or rather 4-weekly; therefore, there are 13 periods–measles data from page 59 allows the reconstruction of these quantities (see online Glasgow measles). It is not quite clear how the 4-weekly errors are pooled. In any case, Soper finds that the following function appears to fit the observed error (i.e. difference between simple model and Glasgow data) well:

$$k_\theta = \frac{1}{10}\cos\theta - \frac{1}{10}\cos 2\theta. \tag{3.27}$$

As mentioned before, θ represents months 1 through 12 (or four week periods 1 through 13). As the period of the function, which is displayed in Fig. 7, is the full year and thus 12 months (13 4-week periods), the value of θ_m is $\theta_m = \frac{m2\pi}{12}$ or, if there are 13 4-week periods in the year, $\theta_w = \frac{w2\pi}{13}$. Soper comments on that seasonal "infectivity" function that

> *"It thus roughly represents changes of concentration, such as are brought about by school and holidays, that are generally held to be answerable in some measure for the changes in infectivity." (p. 42, end of fourth paragraph)*

This would still, to a large extent, be a modern view of the seasonal factors driving transmission of a directly transmitted disease such as measles.

Soper then extensively discusses two multi-year "synthetic" (= simulated) epidemics that are generated by the iterative model represented in Eqs. (13) and (14) and that are shown in Figs. 9 and 10.

Question 3.p

Under the description of Fig. 10 (p. 46, approx. middle of page) he states that

> *"[...] the fifth and sixth years very nearly reproduce the composite picture of the Glasgow epidemics '01–'12, and in particular the years '01–'02, '11–'12 (see Fig. 11)."*

Comment on the significance of the observation that the simulated epidemic in two years closely resembles the composite Glasgow data.

Refinement of the model

On the following pages, Soper endeavors to refine the model by a number of steps. Some of these steps are quite obscure, but, I am confident, justified, at least in the scientific historic context. For example, he proposes to adjust the "known" numbers of susceptibles by the constant A (middle of p. 49). By "known" I am referring to the numbers calculated from the supposed equilibrium number of susceptibles, the subtraction of cases and the addition of the assumed monthly "influx". The rationale for this adjustment is not clearly laid out. He also tries to get a better estimate of the accession rate (addition of susceptibles) by the examination of annual measles case numbers during 1906 through 1916, when the annual measles incidence of Glasgow seemed relatively constant (p. 48). The idea behind this is the assumption that the population is in demographic and epidemic equilibrium such that the sum of all cases must equal the sum of newly added susceptibles. He also investigates different choices for the generation time (one week, two weeks, and four weeks) (p. 50) and, finally, a "non-parametric" method of estimating the season factor (pp. 51 and 52). Other statistical considerations are given. Some of these procedures are not easy to understand, but because the details seem of minor importance I will not try to elucidate them here. Yet, the remainder of the main part of the paper (bottom of p. 52 through p. 58) reveals Soper's insight and, to some extent, awareness of the limitations of his modeling approach.

Appendix 3.A

I will finish my analysis of the chapter with "Appendix 3.A" in which an ordinary differential equation (often abbreviated ODE) transmission model is developed with the purpose of investigating the effect of a deviation from the "instant" hypothesis according to which those infected, after their incubation period (again, according to modern terminology, this should be latent period) instantaneously dispose themselves of their infectious power by infecting all secondary cases in an instant. As we have seen, this model results in stable periodicity without any dampening. Soper now investigates the consequences of assuming a continuous-time model according to which constant infectiousness persists from the time of infection to recovery especially on the periodicity. Here is the model:

$$\frac{dx}{dt} = a - a\frac{x}{as}\frac{y}{a\tau}, \tag{3.28}$$

$$\frac{dy}{dt} = a\frac{x}{as}\frac{y}{a\tau} - a\frac{y}{a\tau}. \tag{3.29}$$

A few general explanations:

1. As this is a continuous-time model, events do not happen in discrete steps (earlier in the paper, this framework is referred to as "instant" hypothesis); This is both true for transmission and recovery events.

2. The all events occur at specific rates; "recovery", i.e. the process of losing infectiousness, for example, occurs at a rate $\frac{1}{\tau}$. Remember that in this context, we are not interested in what we colloquially refer to as "recovery"; we only care about infectiousness! The mean duration of infectiousness therefore is τ; this is a property of the exponential distribution: The mean time to event is the inverse of the rate at which the event occurs.
3. The parameter a is still the "accession" rate, i.e. the rate at which new susceptibles are generated.
4. "Equilibrium" is reached when the rate at which new cases are generated remains constant–that can only be when that rate equals the rate at which susceptibles are added to the population. The number of susceptibles will then be $x^* = as$ and the number of infecteds will be $y^* = a\tau$.
5. The term $a\frac{x}{as}\frac{y}{a\tau}$ in Eqs. (3.28) and (3.29) can be simplified to $\frac{xy}{as\tau}$, which would make it clear (at least after we worked through the following chapters, especially Chap. 4) that $\frac{1}{as\tau}$ is the transmission parameter. Soper presumably chose the more complicated notation to contain the equilibrium values for x and y. Similarly, the term $a\frac{y}{a\tau}$ in Eq. (3.29) can be simplified to $y\frac{1}{\tau}$; this is the rate by which y decreases due to recovery: the per-capita recovery rate, applied to all those y prone to recover from infectiousness.

Question 3.q

Soper remarks regarding the recovery process that

> *"Let us also suppose that this may happen with equal chance dt at any instant, so that τ is the mean "life" in the infecting condition". (p. 60, second paragraph)*

Think about whether, and if so, how this statement relates to the model represented in Eqs. (3.28) and (3.29).

Question 3.r

Derive the quantities x^* and y^*.

Soper then parametrizes the discrete version of the model (the discrete version of an ODE model is called *difference equation model*) using Hamer's London data

$$
\begin{aligned}
x_{k+1} &= x_k + 2{,}200 - \frac{x_k y_k}{300{,}000}, \\
y_{k+1} &= y_k + \frac{x_k y_k}{300{,}000} - \frac{y_k}{2}.
\end{aligned}
$$

The notation of Eqs. (ii) in the Appendix is, from today's perspective, unusual, and I therefore took the liberty to "amend" it to explicitly reflect the recursive nature of the model. The model is implemented in the online Supplement for Appendix 3.A. Soper then states that

> *"Damping down of oscillations is therefore to be expected on the theory that infecting power, instead of being "instant" after an "interval" is prolonged from the time infection was taken for a "chance" space of time." (top of page 61)*

Again, there is no room for chance in the current model, but what Soper refers to is the fact that, according the model, a small proportion of those infected remain infected for a very long time, as only a part $\frac{1}{\tau}$ of them will recover per time step–there will always remain a "left-over" portion. The mathematical explanation of why the "instant" model is periodic, without decrease in amplitude, but the current model shows damped oscillation is difficult and not the focus here.

However, Soper endeavors to explore the problem of periodicity and of the damping factor using a model of "small fractional departures in x and y from their steady-state values", $x^* = as$ and $y^* = a\tau$ by the amounts u and v, respectively:

$$\frac{x}{as} = 1 + u \tag{3.30}$$

at equilibrium, $u = 0$ and $\frac{x^*}{as} = 1 - u$ represents those small deviations from equilibrium. Similarly,

$$\frac{y}{a\tau} = 1 + v. \tag{3.31}$$

To convert Eqs. (3.28) and (3.29) into equations for u and v, we have to figure out how $\frac{du}{dt}$ relates to $\frac{dx}{dt}$ (and the same for v and y):

$$\begin{aligned}
\frac{x}{as} &= 1+u, \\
x &= as + asu \text{ (multiply both sides with } as\text{, which is a constant)}, \\
\frac{dx}{dt} &= \frac{d(as+asu)}{dt} \text{ (take derivative with respect to } t\text{, both sides)} \\
&= \frac{d(as)}{dt} + \frac{d(asu)}{dt} \text{ (do some algebra)} \\
&= 0 + as\frac{du}{dt} \text{ (use general properties of derivatives)}, \\
\frac{dx}{dt} &= as\frac{du}{dt}.
\end{aligned}$$

The equivalent can be done for v and y to obtain $\frac{dy}{dt} = a\tau\frac{dv}{dt}$.

We can now rewrite Eqs. (3.28) and (3.29) as equations for u and v:

$$\begin{aligned}
as\frac{du}{dt} &= a - a(1+u)(1+v) \text{ (substitute } u \text{ for } \frac{x}{as} \text{ and } v \text{ for } \frac{y}{a\tau}\text{)}, \\
s\frac{du}{dt} &= 1 - 1 - u - v - uv \text{ (divide both sides by } a \text{ and multiply out)},
\end{aligned}$$

$$
\begin{aligned}
s\frac{du}{dt} &= -u - v \\
&\quad \text{(simplify and ignore } uv\text{–see p. 61, just above equations)}, \qquad (3.32) \\
a\tau\frac{dv}{dt} &= a(1+u)(1+v) - av \\
&\quad \text{(divide both sides by } a \text{ and multiply left-hand side out)}, \\
\tau\frac{dv}{dt} &= (1+u)(1+v) - v \\
&\quad \text{(divide both sides by } a \text{ and multiply left-hand side out)} \\
&= u + v - v \text{ (multiply out, ignore product } uv\text{)}, \\
\tau\frac{dv}{dt} &= v. \qquad (3.33)
\end{aligned}
$$

Now, Eq. (3.32) can be transformed into a second order homogeneous differential equation which will be used to figure out the period and damping of the system:

$$
\begin{aligned}
s\frac{du}{dt} &= -u - v, \\
s\frac{du}{dt} + u + v &= 0 \text{ (add } -u - v \text{ to both sides)}, \\
\frac{du}{dt} + \frac{1}{s}u + \frac{1}{s}v &= 0 \text{ (divide both sides by } s\text{)}, \\
\frac{d^2u}{dt^2} + \frac{1}{s}\frac{du}{dt} + \frac{1}{s}\frac{dv}{dt} &= 0 \text{ (take derivative with respect to } t\text{)}, \\
\frac{d^2u}{dt^2} + \frac{1}{s}\frac{du}{dt} + \frac{1}{s\tau}u &= 0 \text{ (substitute left-hand side of Eq. (3.33) for } \frac{dv}{dt}\text{)}. \qquad (3.34)
\end{aligned}
$$

Note that, dividing Eq. (3.33) by τ, we obtain $\frac{dv}{dt} = \frac{1}{\tau}v$, thus τ in the second denominator (left-hand side) of (3.34).

The solution to Eq. (3.34) is (as can be seen in many texts on differential equations) is of the form

$$u(t) = c_1 \exp(\lambda t)\cos(\mu t) + c_2 \exp(\lambda t)\sin(\mu t).$$

Here, $\lambda = -\frac{1}{2s}$ and $\mu = \sqrt{1 - \frac{\tau}{4s}\frac{1}{\sqrt{s\tau}}}$ (see Eq. (iii) on p. 61). The period of that system therefore is

$$\frac{2\pi\sqrt{s\tau}}{\sqrt{1 - \frac{\tau}{4s}}}. \qquad (3.35)$$

Also see the discussion of the relationship between the argument of the cosine function and the period on page 44.

The damping factor is $\exp(-\frac{t}{2s})$. If we calculate the period based on expression (3.35), we obtain

$$\begin{aligned}\frac{2\pi\sqrt{s\tau}}{\sqrt{1-\frac{\tau}{4s}}} &= \frac{2\times 3.14\times\sqrt{68.2\times 2}}{\sqrt{1-\frac{2}{4\times 68.2}}}\\ &= 73.62.\end{aligned}$$

Plugging this value into the expression for the damping factor $\exp(-\frac{t}{2s})$ and using the value of 68.2 for s, we calculate it as 0.582–this is the *per-period damping factor*. Soper concludes his paper as follows:

> *"For the case, studied arithmetically, in which $\tau = 2$, $s = 68.2$ and first peak was threefold, the period was found 77 weeks in place of 73.7, calculated for small oscillations, and the second peak was found to be 0.80 of the first peak in place of 0.58 so calculated." (end of p. 61)*

Question 3.s

What do you think of Soper's somber assessment of his method to calculate the period of this system, basically admitting to an error of almost 18% (58% *calculated* vs. 80% *observed* damping)?

The discussion

Soper "read" his paper to the *Royal Statistical Society*, i.e. he presented it to this group. This presentation was followed by a discussion which is interesting to read, especially from a historical perspective. But I will only present two of my favorite passages. Dr. Crookshank, a practicing physician, before embarking into a lengthy tirade of annihilating criticism states that

> *"He had the profoundest admiration for the mathematical part of the paper; truly, he did not understand anything about it, and perhaps that was why he had such an admiration for it. But he had to confess to a profound distrust of statistical method on all occasions excepting when applied to the examination of a particular theory, or of particular data." (p. 64)*

Of course, his profound lack of understanding is evidenced by referring to Soper's work as "statistical method"–there was hardly any statistical consideration involved. Crookshank's views, by the way, left little scientific impact.

Professor Greenwood who did not share Dr. Crookshank's abysmal view of Soper's paper

> *"suggested that Mr. Soper's plan in this paper of taking an epidemiological hypothesis, expressing that hypothesis arithmetically and determining how nearly it described the observations of others, was the one way in which one could hope to render more precise the description of epidemiological phenomena." (p. 69)*

He therefore conveys profound understanding and a modern conception of mathematical epidemiology that was ahead of his time.

Appendix 3.B Answers

3.a It appears that the discussion of the "stability of type" can only be understood from a historical perspective (see, e.g. [4]). When Hamer gave his lecture, the microbiological revolution, brought on by Robert Koch's and Louis Pasteur's discoveries, was still young. The resulting "typology" of infectious diseases was still very much in flux. To me, these introductory paragraphs are hard to fully appreciate; I interpret them as a justification for the discussion of disease periodicity that is designed to prove the etiological unity of measles: it is only one stable organism and fluctuations in the number susceptible that can produce periodic incidence!

3.b Being an "obligatory parasite" is of great importance here as it implies that the risk of infection is independent of an environmental reservoir, but is proportional to the number of individuals that are infectious. This is a simplified statement which will be revisited throughout the book. Full immunity after infection, especially in the case of measles, is important because it implies that susceptibility to infection can be lost, but not regained. Note that there is no one single right answer.

3.c Maternal anti-measles antibodies are transplacentally transferred to the fetus. These antibodies persist to up to a year and induce passive immunity to the measles virus (see, e.g., [3]). However, those insusceptible infants would later become susceptible, adding to the influx of susceptible individuals. The temporary immunity of infants due to maternal antibodies would therefore not lead to a decrease in the influx of susceptibles.

3.d "One infects one" means that there is no increase or decrease of the number of cases. This will be the case where the tangent to the curve is horizontal which is the case at the peak and the nadir of the epidemic curve depicted in "Fig. 7". Mathematically, this corresponds to a (local[12]) maximum and minimum which are points on the curve where the first derivative of the curve is zero.
We have not yet acquired the mathematical tools to derive the fact that the number of susceptibles is equal at A and K, but the fact can be derived "heuristically" (without mathematical rigor).

3.e The area ADB represents the rate at which more measles cases (= susceptibles depleted) than susceptibles are produced, starting with the peak A. Note that, as there are more susceptible removed than added, there must be fewer susceptibles at B than at A. As the system, by assumption, is in equilibrium, such that the total number in the population remains constant, the number of susceptibles must be the same at A and K; therefore, the excess removal of susceptibles (ADB) must equal the excess addition of susceptibles (BHK).

3.f If the number of susceptibles is the only factor determining the number of secondary cases derived from one case and if x is the number of susceptibles at Z (and A and K) and if there are 180,000 susceptibles in C then one case at C must infect

[12] Local refers to the fact that the minimum/maximum may not be universal; this is especially true for a periodic epidemic curved as discussed here.

$\frac{180{,}000}{150{,}000} = \frac{6}{5} = \frac{2{,}400}{2{,}000}$ cases; the equation therefore is inconsistent with the constructed "reality". His conclusion that, therefore, the epidemic curve must be asymmetrical demonstrates deep insight into transmission dynamics: Typical "epidemic curves" displaying the incidence of cases over time in fact exhibit this asymmetry, the ascending leg being less steep than the descending one. This insight is, however, not well communicated and the fact that the logically inconsistent equation is displayed may betray some level of unclarity of Hamer's thinking. Critical reading will habitually unearth minor flaws which, however, should never detract from author's main accomplishments!

3.g In the case of influenza, Hamer appears to attribute the "slackening" in the increase of cases of influenza to the fact that the "specially exposed" people are removed first without making any reference to the depletion of susceptibles which seemed to explain so much of the periodicity of measles. The depletion of the specially exposed also, in Hamer's view, explains the slow decline in incidence ("trailing epidemic"). The question to what extent "influenza" exhibited *persistency of type*; the disease manifestation of influenza is notoriously of low specificity, i.e. agents (especially viruses) cause diseases clinically indistinguishable to disease caused by influenza viruses. Influenza viruses were identified in the 1930s; it is likely that "trailing epidemics" of London reflected incidence fluctuations of a conglomerate of acute respiratory illness of different causes.

3.h Soper refers to the instant where the "infecting power" of the primary case is concentrated. This model, i.e. the assumption that all secondary cases due to one case are generated in one instant, simplifies the mathematical discussion....

3.i Different justifications can be given. The most intuitive one is this. Assume that the population of size N is wholly susceptible and that, in that context, n cases result from the index case. This implies that there were n contacts that led to infection (infectious contacts). Now assume that only x susceptibles remain in the population, i.e. a proportion $\frac{x}{N}$ remains susceptible. The probability that a (potentially) infectious contact of a case is with a susceptible person is $\frac{x}{N}$. Therefore, instead of n cases, $\frac{nx}{N}$ are expected to result from one case. We can write

$$\frac{nx}{N} = q.$$

Let m denote the number of susceptibles for which a case results in exactly *one* secondary case. We can then write

$$\frac{nm}{N} = 1.$$

If we then divide the left- and right-hand sides of the first equation by the left- and right-hand sides of the second equation, we obtain:

$$\frac{\frac{nx}{N}}{\frac{nm}{N}} = \frac{q}{1}.$$

Simplifying we get

$$\frac{x}{m} = q$$

which completes the proof that the number of secondary cases per case is the ratio of the number of susceptibles to the number of susceptibles at "equilibrium" ("one makes one").

3.j This directly follows from the equality $m = s\,a$ given at the bottom of page 37. Remember that this was introduced for rendering the "synthetic"–today we would say: *simulated*–epidemic independent of the absolute population size. As we will see in later chapters, this is not necessarily the most straightforward approach to that goal.

3.k The two implementations (online Supplement) of the synthetic epidemic can be described as follows: At the peak of the epidemic, when the simulation is started, there are $z(0) = 4{,}000$ infections per unit of time; these are derived from the equilibrium number of susceptibles, $x(0) = 40{,}000$. For the next time step, these 4,000 infections have to be subtracted from the susceptibles, which are augmented by $a = 1{,}000$:

$$
\begin{aligned}
x(1) &= x(0) - z(0) + a, \\
z(1) &= z(0)\frac{x(1)}{m},
\end{aligned}
$$

or, more generally,

$$
\begin{aligned}
x(t+1) &= x(t) - z(t) + a, \\
z(t+1) &= z(t)\frac{x(t+1)}{m}.
\end{aligned}
$$

3.l As $z = a\exp(u) = z_{t-1}\frac{x_t}{s\,a}$, we can solve for u:

$$
\begin{aligned}
a\exp(u) &= z_{t-1}\frac{x_t}{s\,a}, \\
\exp(u) &= z_{t-1}\frac{x_t}{s\,a^2} \text{ (after dividing both sides by } a\text{)}, \\
u &= \log\left(z_{t-1}\frac{x_t}{s\,a^2}\right) \text{ (after taking the natural logarithm of both sides)}.
\end{aligned}
$$

The last line constitutes the answer to the question.

3.m We can calculate u using the formula in the answer to Question 3.l, for example, in the spreadsheet that contains our "synthetic epidemic". To justify that exercise, we have to assume that the length of a time step is τ, the incubation period of the diseases. Using the numbers in the spreadsheet for z, x, s, and a, we see that, at least at the epidemic peak, it is not "small" (larger than 1).

3.n The two expressions for u are not equal, but asymptotically equivalent with respect to their period. By "asymptotically" I meant that, as Soper states, if the epidemics are *small*. We can play around with this, for example, in the spreadsheet (online Supplement), making $z(0)$ small, say 1,200. The periods of the two functions then very closely match. Note that $z(0)$ cannot be smaller than a (the renewal constant of the population) because otherwise the assumption that z_0 is an infection number at the peak is no longer met (the number of infections increases because the number of susceptibles is increasing, and we thus are not starting our simulation at the equilibrium value m).

3.o Soper was mistaken by his guess. When there are small oscillations, with 1010 cases at peak, the period of the epidemics is 28 units (incubation periods). Increasing peak cases to 2010 leaves the period at 28; with 3010 peak cases, the period is lengthened to 30 (7.1% increase), and with 4010 cases the period is 32 (6.7% increase). Note that the period is found from the sequence u1 (column I in the spreadsheet) by identifying the first maximum and the corresponding "time".

3.p The similarity between the simulated epidemic of Fig. 10 and the composite Glasgow data (six biennia added by month in two-year period) shows, in fact, remarkable resemblance. However, I believe that similarity is entirely coincidental and irrelevant, i.e. without any deeper meaning. Such comparison might be "meaningful" if the epidemic process had solid 2-year periodicity and the summation of the data would reduce sampling variation (the variability which is only due to random fluctuations). Examining the measles data in Fig. 11, even when restricted to the six biennia, there does not seem to be "clean" periodicity, even though the large peaks are quite regular.

3.q Chance, of course, has no place in this model as this is a deterministic model (just like the discrete time model was). However, rates such as $\frac{1}{\tau}$ are key components in such models. In a stochastic context, where chance plays a role, a rate can be defined like Soper does in his remark.

3.r These quantities can be explained as follows: At equilibrium, Eqs. (3.28) and (3.29) become

$$0 = a - a\frac{x^*}{as}\frac{y^*}{a\tau}, \quad (3.36)$$

$$0 = a\frac{x^*}{a\tau} - a\frac{y^*}{a\tau}. \quad (3.37)$$

At equilibrium, both equations equal 0 because neither x nor y changes. This is a system of two equations in two unknowns and can therefore be solved:

1. Add both equations to get

$$\begin{aligned} 0 &= a - a\frac{y^*}{a\tau}, \\ a &= a\frac{y^*}{a\tau} \\ &= \frac{y^*}{\tau} \text{ (cancel } a \text{ in fraction)}, \\ y^* &= a\tau \text{ (multiply both sides with } \tau). \end{aligned}$$

2. Plug the solution of y^* into (3.36):

$$
\begin{aligned}
0 &= a - a\frac{x^*}{as}\frac{a\tau}{a\tau},\\
0 &= a - \frac{x^*}{s} \text{ (simplify)},\\
x^* &= as \text{ (add } \frac{x^*}{s} \text{ to both sides, multiply with } s).
\end{aligned}
$$

3.s Soper actually makes a computational error: He compares the per-period damping factor, 0.58, with the size of the second peak (5,944) relative to the first peak (6,500), which is 91.6% rather than 80% as stated in the quote. However, the damping applies only to the oscillations from the mean or eventual equilibrium y^*. So while the deviation of the first peak from the equilibrium value is $6{,}500 - 4{,}400 = 2{,}100$, the calculated per-period damping value of 0.582 would mean the next peak's deviation would be $2{,}100 \times 0.582 = 1222.2$ such that the next peak would be $4{,}000 + 1222.2 = 5222.2$, or 80.3% of the first peak. So the error is 12.3% rather than 18%. Note that the model for u and v is not just a model for small oscillations; it is actually the identical model as the one for x and y. The error, presumably, stems from ignoring the uv product.

Appendix 3.C Supplementary material

Supplementary material related to this chapter can be found online at http://dx.doi.org/10.1016/B978-0-12-802260-3.00003-1.

References

[1] H. Soper, The interpretation of periodicity in disease prevalence, Journal of the Royal Statistical Society (1929) 34–73.
[2] W.H. Hamer, The Milroy Lectures on Epidemic Disease in England: The Evidence of Variability and of Persistency of Type, Bedford Press, 1906.
[3] H. Sato, P. Albrecht, D.W. Reynolds, S. Stagno, F.A. Ennis, Transfer of measles, mumps, and rubella antibodies from mother to infant: its effect on measles, mumps, and rubella immunization, American Journal of Diseases of Children 133 (12) (1979) 1240–1243.
[4] B.A. Whitelegge, The Milroy lectures on changes of type in epidemic diseases: delivered at the Royal College of Physicians, British Medical Journal 1 (1678) (1893) 393, BMJ Group.

W.O. Kermack and A.G. McKendrick: A seminal contribution to the mathematical theory of epidemics (1927)

4

Contents

4.1 Introduction

This chapter discusses the likely most influential contribution to the mathematical modeling of infectious diseases which preceded Soper's presentation of disease periodicity [8] by two years [5]. The paper is cited in uncountable papers for the "Kermack–McKendrick" model, but it seems likely that many of these citations are "mechanistic", i.e. they cite because other papers cited the work etc. Unlike in the preceding papers [2,4,8], the mathematical formalism used seems largely consistent and will likely provide far less opportunity for "criticism" than some of the previous works. We will follow most of the mathematical arguments up to the climax of the classical "SIR" model for which this paper is usually cited. The paper has subheadings, such as "General theory" etc., but its structure may be better reflected by inconspicuously placed numbers from (1) to (13). Some of these sections, the beginning of which sometimes, but not always coincides with the start of a titled section, are more relevant than others, and we will treat some of them only summarily. The introduction section of this paper, prefaced by the number (1), broadly outlines its background and purpose, referencing only the work of Ross and Hudson [6,7] which, in this paper, is "[...] carried to a further stage, and it is considered from a point of view which is in one sense more general." Some of Ross's work will be discussed in the following chapter.

A Historical Introduction to Mathematical Modeling of Infectious Diseases. DOI: 10.1016/B978-0-12-802260-3.00004-3

Question 4.a

At the bottom of p. 701 it is stated that

> *"Two of the reasons commonly put forward as accounting for the termination of an epidemic, are (1) that the susceptible individuals have all been removed, and (2) that during the course of the epidemic the virulence of the causative organism has gradually decreased."*

Comment on this statement in the light of what we have learned so far.

4.2 General theory: (2) through (7)

4.2.1 (2): The infection process in discrete time

Kermack & McKendrick open their theoretical argument using a discrete time model of disease transmission with the time step constituting the time unit. The number of individuals ill or, more significantly, infectious at time step t is denoted by y_t. Infections happen at the transition between two time intervals, and infectious individuals at time t are characterized by the number of time steps since they have been infected and are denoted by $v_{t,\theta}$; θ represents the number of intervals since infection. The newly infected individuals are denoted by v_t which is equivalent to $v_{t,0}$. Furthermore, infection naturally is assumed to enter the community not *de novo*, but to start with the infection of a member or members of the population who has/have acquired infection from an "external" source. Consistent with the notation, the number of index cases (i.e. infections that start outbreak) is denoted by $v_{0,0} = y_0 = v_0$. With progression of time by one step, this number progresses to $v_{1,1}$ (see figure on p. 703 in [5]). As all new infections start with $\theta = 0$, i.e. as $v_{t,0}$ if infection is acquired at time t, $v_{t+1,\theta+1}$ cannot be bigger than $v_{t,\theta}$, but has to be smaller. Attrition of infections is referred to as "removal" which can happen as the result of death or simply loosing infectiousness. The removal process is parameterized by ψ_θ which is the proportion removed at the end of stage θ. Note that ψ has to be positive and not bigger than one, i.e. $\psi \in [0, 1]$ (for readers not familiar with this notation it reads: "ψ lies in the range from (including) zero to (including) one"). Accordingly, the proportion of infections persisting to the next interval is $1 - \psi_\theta$. The number of infections $v_{1,1}$ deriving from $v_{0,0}$ is therefore given by the relationship

$$v_{1,1} = v_{0,0} \times (1 - \psi_0).$$

Note that, in Eq. 2 on p. 703 ψ_θ is written as $\psi(\theta)$.

Question 4.b

Given the stated assumptions about ψ, what does this imply for $v_{1,1}$.

Similarly,

$$v_{2,2} = v_{0,0}(1 - \psi_0)(1 - \psi_1).$$

More concisely, this could be written as

$$v_{2,2} = v_{0,0} \prod_{\theta=0}^{1} (1 - \psi_\theta)$$

and, more generally,

$$v_{t,\theta} = v_{t-\theta,0} \prod_{\theta=0}^{\theta-1} (1 - \psi_\theta).$$

Note that $\psi_\theta v_{t,\theta} = v_{t,\theta} - v_{t+1,\theta+1}$.

> **Question 4.c**
>
> Show that this equality is true.

Conveniently, Kermack and McKendrick introduce the notation

$$\mathbf{B}_\theta = \prod_{\theta=0}^{\theta-1} (1 - \psi_\theta). \tag{4.1}$$

An intuitive interpretation of $\mathbf{B}_\theta$ is the proportion, or probability, to "escape" removal through interval θ after infection.

New infections

As implied by the figure, the number of new infections at the end of time interval t is denoted by $v_t = v_{t,0}$. This equality holds because, by definition, $v_{t,0}$ is the number of subjects who, at the end of interval t have been infected for 0 time intervals. The exception for this is time $t = 0$ when $v_0 = v_{0,0} + y_0$. The need for this exception may not be immediately evident.

> **Question 4.d**
>
> If, instead of removal, the event that occurs with probability θ were to be death, what would be an appropriate term for $\mathbf{B}_\theta$?

The number of new infections in interval t, v_t, must, given our fundamental assumptions regarding the perpetuation of infection, be a function of the current infections.

> **Question 4.e**
>
> We have not, in fact, extensively talked about those referenced "fundamental assumptions". Please list those assumptions that are really fundamental. Like so often, there will not be one single correct answer!

Kermack & McKendrick write (mid-page 703) that

> "*[v_t] must be equal to $x_t \sum_1^t \phi_\theta v_{t,\theta}$*,"

i.e.

$$v_t = x(t) \sum_{\theta=1}^{t} \phi_\theta v_{t,\theta} \tag{4.2}$$

where $x(t)$ denotes the number of subjects still susceptible at time t and ϕ_θ represents the "rate of infectivity at age θ"; here, "age" refers to time since infection. Note that, by assumption, during the time interval when they first appear as infected, individuals $v_{t,0}$ are assumed to be not infectious. This is why summation starts at 1 instead of 0.

Question 4.f

Kermack & McKendrick do not elaborate on the "rate of infectivity", but a clear understanding of this parameter is of great importance. What does the expression for v_t imply for the units of the rate of infectivity?

As the number of susceptibles[1] only changes when susceptibles enter the infectious class, the following expression is given (expression (3))

$$\begin{aligned} x(t) &= N - \sum_0^t v_{t,0} \\ &= N - \sum_0^t v_t - y_0. \end{aligned}$$

The notation here is ambiguous and should, for better clarity, be replaced by

$$x(t) = N - \sum_{s=0}^{t} v_s - y_0.$$

This apparent subtlety is important as the original version of the expression (second line, left-hand) can be translated to "N minus the sum of v_t from $t = 0$ to $t = t$." So t is used as a summation index (in v_t) as well as a limit of the summation (in "sum [...] from $t = 0$ to $t = t$"). The second version of the expression clearly separates the summation index and the limit; this will be even more important and confusion may arise when the time intervals tend to zero and we are dealing with integrals.

[1] The term "susceptibles", or "infectives", etc. clearly is poor use of the English language. However, these terms are commonly used to refer to the *numbers* of susceptible or infectious, respectively.

Question 4.g

In the second line of expression (3), $x(t) = N - \sum_0^t v_t - y_0$. What does this imply for the expression or, more specifically, does this result in a mistake in the expression?

The next expression ((4), bottom p. 703) formulates constraints for x_t, y_t, and z_t:

$$x_t + y_t + z_t = N. \tag{4.3}$$

A *constraint* is a condition that restricts the range, in this case, of the three variables which a priori only have to be positive numbers (real numbers, as implied by the answer to Question 4.a). The variable z_t is introduced here for the first time: it represents the numbers of "removed" (either by recovery or death). The most important characteristics of z_t are that they are neither susceptible nor infectious. The constraint indicates that the variables x_t, y_t, and z_t are forced:

- To be no larger than N, i.e. $x_t, y_t, z_t \leq N$;
- To give a sum of N; this implies that, when two are given the third one is determined. If, e.g. $N = 1000$, $x_t = 900$, $y_t = 10$ then, necessarily, $z_t = 90$.

Expression (4.2) can be written as

$$\begin{aligned} v_t &= x_t \sum_{\theta=1}^{t} \phi_\theta v_{t,\theta} && (4.4) \\ &= x_t \sum_{1}^{t} \phi_\theta \mathrm{B}_\theta v_{t-\theta,0} && (4.5) \\ &= x_t \left(\sum_{1}^{t} \mathrm{A}_\theta v_{t-\theta} + \mathrm{A}_t y_0 \right). && (4.6) \end{aligned}$$

Remember that $v_t = v_{t,0}$ represents the number of new infections during time interval t. To simplify the notation, $\mathrm{A}_\theta = \phi_\theta \mathrm{B}_\theta$.

Question 4.h

Can A_θ, B_θ, and/or C_θ be expressed as probabilities? If yes, do so; if no, explain.

The number of infectious individuals at the end of time interval t, y_t, can be calculated by summing over all those still infectious at time t, i.e. $v_{t,0} = v_0 \mathrm{B}_t$ (infectious since the end of the first interval; having "survived", i.e. escaped "removal" for t time intervals), $v_{t,1} = v_0 \mathrm{B}_{t-1}$, etc. Therefore,

$$y_t = \sum_{\theta=0}^{t} v_{t,\theta} = \sum_{\theta=0}^{t} \mathrm{B}_\theta v_{t-\theta} + \sum_{\theta=0}^{t} \mathrm{B}_t y_0. \tag{4.7}$$

As the number of new infections at the end of interval t must be equal to the difference of the number individuals susceptible at the beginning of the previous interval, x_t, and the next interval, x_{t+1}, we have $v_t = x_t - x_{t+1}$, or

$$-v_t = x_{t+1} - x_t. \tag{4.8}$$

Eq. (4.8) holds because the number of new infections, v_t, must be a positive number; x_{t+1}, however, must be smaller than x_t as the number of susceptibles can only decrease with time–there are, by assumption, neither births nor immigration. The difference $x_{t+1} - x_t$ therefore has to be *negative* and is only due to susceptibles becoming infected (v_t). The difference between x_{t+1} and x_t therefore must correspond in size to v_t, v_t must be a *positive* number and, because $x_{t+1} - x_t$ has to be negative, $x_{t+1} - x_t = -v_t$.

Using Eqs. (4.8) (multiplying both sides by -1) and (4.6), we can therefore write

$$x_{t+1} - x_t = -x_t\left(\sum_1^t \mathrm{A}_\theta v_{t-\theta} + \mathrm{A}_t y_0\right). \tag{4.9}$$

Note that Kermack & McKendrick give the expression for $x_t - x_{t+1}$ (expression (8)). As these discrete-time equations will later be transformed into differential equations, the form used in (4.9) seems better suited because it also expresses the change in x by time, i.e. $\frac{x_{t+\Delta}-x_t}{\Delta}$ when Δ tends to zero.

A corresponding equation can be developed for z_t, the number of removed. That expression is similar in structure to Eq. (4.9), but does not involve x; this makes intuitive sense as the removal process does not involve an interaction with individuals of a different state, but can be viewed as a form of a "decay process"–therefore, that change necessarily has to be non-negative: the number of recovered can only increase (or stay the same):

$$z_{t+1} - z_t = \sum_1^t \mathrm{C}_\theta v_{t-\theta} + \mathrm{C}_t y_0. \tag{4.10}$$

Finally, according to expression (4.3), the sum of the numbers of individuals in each class (susceptible, x, infectious, y, and recovered, z) is always N. This implies that when two of the values are given (e.g. x and y) the third one (e.g. z) is determined. We can use this to state the following about y, the number of infectious:

$$\begin{aligned} x_{t+1} + y_{t+1} + z_{t+1} &= N, \\ y_{t+1} &= N - x_{t+1} - z_{t+1}, \end{aligned} \tag{4.11}$$

and

$$\begin{aligned} x_t + y_t + z_t &= N, \\ y_t &= N - x_t - z_t. \end{aligned} \tag{4.12}$$

By subtracting (4.12) from (4.11), we can obtain the following expression:

$$\begin{aligned} y_{t+1} - y_t &= N - x_{t+1} - z_{t+1} - (N - x_t - z_t) \\ &= N - N - x_{t+1} + x_t - z_{t+1} + z_t \\ &= x_t - x_{t+1} + z_t - z_{t+1} \\ &= x_t \left(\sum_1^t \mathrm{A}_\theta v(t-\theta) + \mathrm{A}_t y_0 \right) \\ &\quad - \left(\sum_1^t \mathrm{C}_\theta v(t-\theta) + \mathrm{C}_t y_0 \right). \end{aligned} \tag{4.13}$$

Eq. (4.10) corresponds to expression (10) in Kermack & McKendrick and is obtained by taking the negative of (4.9) because $x_t - x_{t+1}$ is the negative of $x_{t+1} - x_t$ (see (4.9)) and, for the same reason, the negative of (4.10).

4.2.2 (3): The infection process in continuous time

We are now ready to move on to a continuous-time representation of the system of equations representing the change in the variables x_t, y_t, and z_t. If we let the time step from t to $t+1$ become infinitesimally small, summations ($\sum$) also must be substituted for by integrations ($\int$). Note that, e.g. $\frac{x_{t+1}-x_t}{\Delta t}$ becomes $\frac{dx(t)}{dt}$; before, e.g. in Eq. (4.9), the Δt denominator was omitted because the time step, Δt, was assumed to be of size 1 (most likely one *day*). Even though Kermack & McKendrick continue to use an index notation as in A_θ, I will use a more "modern" version, using a functional equivalent, e.g. $\mathrm{A}(\theta)$ instead of A_θ:

$$\frac{dx(t)}{dt} = -x(t)\left[\int_0^t \mathrm{A}(\theta)v(t-\theta)d\theta + \mathrm{A}(t)y(0)\right], \tag{4.14}$$

$$\begin{aligned} \frac{dy(t)}{dt} &= x(t)\left(\int_0^t \mathrm{A}(\theta)v(t-\theta)d\theta + \mathrm{A}(t)y(0)\right) \\ &\quad - \left(\int_1^t \mathrm{C}(\theta)v(t-\theta)d\theta + \mathrm{C}(t)y(0)\right), \end{aligned} \tag{4.15}$$

$$\frac{dz(t)}{dt} = \int_0^t \mathrm{C}(\theta)v(t-\theta)d\theta + \mathrm{C}(t)y(0). \tag{4.16}$$

Note that, instead of Eq. (4.15), Kermack & McKendrick give, based on their expression (6) (here (4.7)) an expression for $y(t)$:

$$y(t) = \int_0^t \mathrm{B}(\theta)v(t-\theta)d\theta + \mathrm{B}(t)y(0). \tag{4.17}$$

Question 4.i

Consider the parameters A_θ, $B(\theta)$, and $C(\theta)$. We defined them in terms of discrete time steps (see (4.1)). Define continuous-time equivalent definitions for these parameters for the use in Eqs. (4.14), (4.15), and (4.16).

The following mathematical development focuses on Eq. (4.14) rather than (4.15), which would seem more intuitive for a treatment of an epidemic process: $y(t)$, after all, denotes the number[2] of infectious individuals. $x(t)$, however, is a mirror of $v(t)$, the number of *new* infections, as in this model there is no other way than the infection process to change x. Specifically,

$$v(t) = -\frac{x(t)}{dt}. \tag{4.18}$$

Eq. (4.14) can be algebraically transformed as follows:

$$\begin{aligned}
\frac{dx(t)}{dt} &= -x(t)\left[\int_0^t A(\theta)v(t-\theta)d\theta + A(t)y(0)\right] && (4.19)\\
&= -x(t)\left[\int_0^t A(t-\theta)v(\theta)d\theta + A(t)y(0)\right] && (4.20)\\
&= x(t)\left[\int_0^t A(t-\theta)\frac{dx(\theta)}{d\theta}d\theta - A(t)y(0)\right]. && (4.21)
\end{aligned}$$

Question 4.j

Consider the exchange of arguments of A and v from $t-\theta$ to t and *vice versa* in Eq. (4.20). Please explain and justify.

Expression (4.21) can also be written as

$$\begin{aligned}
\frac{dx(t)}{dt} &= x(t)\left[\int_0^t A(t-\theta)\frac{dx(\theta)}{d\theta}d\theta - A(t)y(0)\right],\\
\frac{dx(t)}{dt}\frac{1}{x(t)} &= \int_0^t A(t-\theta)\frac{dx(\theta)}{d\theta}d\theta - A(t)y(0) && (4.22)\\
&\quad \text{(dividing both sides by } x\text{)},\\
\frac{d\ln(x(t))}{dt} &= A(t-\theta)x(\theta)|_0^t - \int_0^t x(\theta)\frac{dA(t-\theta)}{d\theta}d\theta - A(t)y(0). && (4.23)
\end{aligned}$$

Some explanations regarding the "magical" transformation of Eq. (4.22) to (4.23) are in order:

[2] Remember that it is actually a "quantity"–see the answer to Question 4.a.

Left-hand side

First, consider the following equality:

$$\frac{d\ln(x(t))}{dx(t)} = \frac{1}{x(t)},$$

i.e. the derivative of the natural logarithm of x with respect to x is $\frac{1}{x}$. This equality can also be stated as

$$\frac{1}{x(t)} = \frac{d\ln(x(t))}{dx(t)}.$$

Therefore, $\frac{1}{x}$ in the expression $\frac{dx(t)}{dt}\frac{1}{x(t)}$ can be substituted with $\frac{d\ln(x(t))}{dx(t)}$, giving

$$\begin{aligned}\frac{dx(t)}{dt}\frac{1}{x(t)} &= \frac{dx(t)}{dt}\frac{d\ln(x(t))}{dx(t)} \\ &= \frac{d\ln(x(t))}{dt} \quad (dx \text{ cancels}).\end{aligned}$$

Right-hand side

On the right-hand side of the equation, *integration by parts*, an important integration technique, is used. Integration by parts is illustrated by the equation

$$\int u dv = uv - \int v du,$$

or for a definite integral,

$$\int_a^b u dv = uv|_a^b - \int_a^b v du.$$

The integral is transformed into a form that is more easily handled. We applied it to the right-hand side of (4.23), with $u = \mathrm{A}(t-\theta)$ and $v = x(t)$. The right-hand side is then further transformed to

$$\frac{d\ln(x(t))}{dt} = \mathrm{A}(0)x(t) - \mathrm{A}_t x(0) + \int_0^t x(\theta)\mathrm{A}'(t-\theta)d\theta - \mathrm{A}(t)y(0) \tag{4.24}$$

where $\mathrm{A}'(t-\theta) = \frac{d\mathrm{A}(t-\theta)}{d(t-\theta)} = -\frac{d\mathrm{A}(t-\theta)}{d\theta}$.

> **Question 4.k**
>
> Explain the change in sign in the expression for $\mathrm{A}'(t-\theta)$ and thus in front of the integral from (4.23) to (4.24).

As, by definition, $A(0) = 0$, i.e. at the moment for their infection subjects are not infectious, Eq. (4.24) simplifies to

$$\begin{aligned}\frac{d\ln(x(t))}{dt} &= -\mathrm{A}_t x(0) - \mathrm{A}(t)y(0) + \int_0^t x(\theta)\mathrm{A}'(t-\theta)d\theta \\ &= -\mathrm{A}_t(x(0)+y(0)) + \int_0^t x(\theta)\mathrm{A}'(t-\theta)d\theta \\ &= -\mathrm{A}_t N + \int_0^t \mathrm{A}'(\theta)x(t-\theta)d\theta \qquad (4.25)\\ &\quad \text{(because } x(0)+y(0)=N\text{).}\end{aligned}$$

Question 4.I

Explain the exchange of arguments in (4.25) between $\mathrm{A}'(\cdot)$ (from $t-\theta$ to θ) and $x(\cdot)$ (from θ to $t-\theta$).

Kermack & McKendrick conclude

> *"We have not been able to solve this equation in such a way as to give x in terms of t as an explicit function." (p. 705, after Eq. (16))*

In the following sections, (4) and (5), Kermack & McKendrick attempt to find recursive solutions to these equations; whether they succeed, I am not completely convinced. However, this part of the paper is of less relevance. Systems of differential equations are not routinely solved numerically–we will see that later in this book. These paragraphs are, at least to me, somewhat obscure. The mathematical argument is tedious at times, with little guidance from the authors. Mathematically more seasoned readers may have less trouble with these passages than myself. However, I believe that some of the premises are unsound as I will explain in Appendix 4.A.

4.2.3 (6): The proportion infected

Returning to Eq. (4.14),

$$\begin{aligned}\frac{dx(t)}{dt} &= -x(t)\left[\int_0^t \mathrm{A}(\theta)v(t-\theta)d\theta + \mathrm{A}(t)y(0)\right], \\ -\frac{d\ln(x(t))}{dt} &= \int_0^t \mathrm{A}(\theta)v(t-\theta)d\theta + \mathrm{A}(t)y(0) \qquad (4.26)\\ &\quad \text{(see expression (4.23)).}\end{aligned}$$

Both sides of the equation are then integrated with respect to t, i.e.

$$-\int_0^\infty \frac{d\ln(x(t))}{dt}dt = \int_0^\infty \int_0^t \mathrm{A}(\theta)v(t-\theta)d\theta dt + \int_0^\infty \mathrm{A}(t)y(0)dt. \qquad (4.27)$$

The reason for that operation is not explicitly stated by Kermack & McKendrick, but, reminding ourselves of the meaning of Eq. (4.23), it becomes obvious: That equation describes the change in susceptibles, x, over time. So $\frac{dx(t)}{dt}$ is a function of time. If we integrate that function over time, we will therefore obtain the numbers susceptible up to a specific time. Eq. (4.23), however, describes the change in $\ln(x(t))$ which does not make intuitive sense. It will, however, produce a relevant result.

The integration of Eq. (4.27) does, at first, seem somewhat obscure. However, again we can use the following property of a convolution integral:

$$\int_0^\infty \int_0^t f(\theta)g(t-\theta)d\theta dt = \int_0^\infty f(t)dt \int_0^\infty g(t)dt. \tag{4.28}$$

Question 4.m

Verify this property for the discrete case, i.e. by replacing the integrations with summations and therefore using discrete instead of continuous time.

Eq. (4.27) can therefore be stated as

$$\ln\left(\frac{x(0)}{x(\infty)}\right) = \int_0^\infty \mathrm{A}(\theta)d\theta \int_0^t v(t)dt + \int_0^\infty \mathrm{A}(t)y(0)dt. \tag{4.29}$$

An explanation may be in order regarding this equation: The left-hand side is explained by the fact that

$$\begin{aligned} -\int_0^\infty \frac{d\ln(x(t))}{dt}dt &= -\int_0^\infty d\ln(x(t)) \\ &= -\ln(x(t))|_0^\infty \\ &= \ln(x(t))|_\infty^0 \\ &= \ln\left(\frac{x(0)}{x(\infty)}\right). \end{aligned}$$

Be reminded that $\mathrm{B}(t) = \exp - \int_0^t \psi(s)ds$ is the "survival" probability (i.e. not recovering from infection) up to time t after infection and $\mathrm{A}(t) = \phi(t)\mathrm{B}(t)$ is the "infection pressure" exerted by an infectious individual at time t, conditional on remaining infected up to that point.

Letting $\mathrm{A} = \int_0^\infty \mathrm{A}(t)dt$ and making use of the relationship (4.18), $v(t) = -\frac{dx}{dt}$, and thus (integrating both sides with respect to time, from 0 to infinity):

$$\int_0^\infty v(t)dt = -\int_0^\infty \frac{dx}{dt}dt = x(0) - x(\infty). \tag{4.30}$$

The left-most quantity is the number of subjects infected over the course of the epidemic: Infection is the only way to leave the class of susceptibles; therefore, the difference between the susceptibles at the outset to the susceptibles left over from the epidemic must be the total number of infections. That same number must be obtained by adding up–or, rather, integrating over–all new infections ($v(\cdot)$). Using these two substitutions in (4.29) gives

$$\begin{aligned}\ln\left(\frac{x(0)}{x(\infty)}\right) &= \mathrm{A}\left(x(0)-x(\infty)\right)+\mathrm{A}y(0)\\ &= \mathrm{A}\left(x(0)-x(\infty)+y(0)\right)\\ &= \mathrm{A}\left(N-x(\infty)\right). \qquad (4.31)\end{aligned}$$

Kermack & McKendrick then define

$$p=\ln\left(\frac{N-x(\infty)}{N}\right) \qquad (4.32)$$

which is the proportion eventually infected and, by solving (4.32) for $x(\infty)$, obtain the following expression for $x(\infty)$, i.e. $x(\infty)=N(1-p)$. Substituting this expression in the right-hand side expression (4.31), the following expression is obtained:

$$-\ln\left(\frac{1-p}{1-\frac{y(0)}{N}}\right)=\mathrm{A}Np. \qquad (4.33)$$

Note that $-\ln\left(\frac{x(\infty)}{x(0)}\right)=\ln\left(\frac{x(0)}{x(\infty)}\right)$. Also, $x(0)=N-y(0)$ so that

$$\begin{aligned}-\ln\left(\frac{x(\infty)}{x(0)}\right) &= -\ln\left(\frac{N(1-p)}{N-y(0)}\right)\\ &= -\ln\left(\frac{1-p}{1-\frac{y(0)}{N}}\right) \text{ (Dividing numerator and denominator by } N\text{).}\end{aligned}$$

While Eq. (4.33) does not allow us to calculate the proportion of eventually infected directly, this equation will be used later.

A similar rationale as the one used for analyzing Eq. (4.19) is then used for Eq. (4.15) to give rise to the following expression:

$$\int_0^\infty y(t)dt=Np\int_0^\infty \mathrm{B}(\theta)d\theta. \qquad (4.34)$$

Question 4.n

Derive expression (4.34) from (4.17) using a similar logic that was used to analyze Eq. (4.19).

"Thus", Kermack & McKendrick write after Eq. (4.34), "$\int_0^\infty \mathrm{B}(\theta)d\theta$ is the average case duration." The reason for that is the following: The left-hand side of the equation, $\int_0^\infty y(t)dt$, integrates over the number infected over time. The result of that operation is a cumulative "infectious time", i.e. the sum[3] of times of infectiousness of all infected individuals. If we divide that sum by all individuals who eventually become infected,

[3] This is an analogy because we are not dealing with individuals–see the answer to Question 4.a.

which is Np, we get the mean time of infectiousness. Returning to Eq. (4.34), we see that if we divide both sides by Np, we get

$$\frac{\int_0^\infty y(t)dt}{Np} = \int_0^\infty \mathrm{B}(\theta)d\theta.$$

On the left-hand side we have, as we have just seen, the mean infectiousness time and on the right-hand side $\int_0^\infty \mathrm{B}(\theta)d\theta$; this is exactly what Kermack & McKendrick state.

4.3 Special cases: (8) through (13)

4.3.1 (10): The "Kermack & McKendrick model"

In the following section (7), Kermack & McKendrick discuss the problem of the "estimation" of the infectivity and removal rates from observable data; the quotes around *estimation* emphasize the fact that this is not a method of statistical estimation, but a method of solving a certain type of integral equation proposed by the Russian Fock [3]. The next part of the paper, entitled *Special Cases*, is in its first two sections (8) & (9) devoted to the "A.–*The earlier stages of an epidemic in a large population*". These passages are mathematically difficult without providing deeper insight into the general problems dealt with here. Instead, I will move on to part "B.–*Constant Rates*" which considers a special case of Eqs. (4.14), (4.15), and (4.16) in which the infection and removal parameters, κ and l, respectively, are constant. This is the central part of the paper which likely also is the basis for its fame. The model, as shown in the paper:

$$\frac{dx}{dt} = -\kappa xy, \tag{4.35}$$

$$\frac{dy}{dt} = \kappa xy - ly, \tag{4.36}$$

$$\frac{dz}{dt} = ly. \tag{4.37}$$

Note that I reverted to the original notation of the paper and dropped the time index ($\frac{dx}{dt}$ instead of $\frac{dx(t)}{dt}$). The transmission parameter, $\phi(t)$, now is constant and denoted κ, and the removal parameter, $\psi(t)$, now is the constant l.

Question 4.o

Characterize the two parameters, κ and l, i.e. explain them and talk about "reasonable" values.

To briefly summarize the "meaning" of these simple, yet fundamental equations (4.35), (4.36), and (4.37):

κxy represents the rate of transfer of *susceptible* individuals to the *infectious* class;
yl represents the transfer of *infectious* individuals to the *removed* class.

Question 4.p

Solve Eqs. (4.35), (4.36), and (4.37) numerically, using any tool at your disposal, except for software specifically designed for dynamic systems modeling (e.g. Berkeley Madonna). Use the values found in answer to Question 4.o.

As $x + y + z = N$, and therefore $y = N - x - z$, Eq. (4.37) can be written as

$$\frac{dz}{dt} = l(N - x - z). \tag{4.38}$$

Dividing Eq. (4.35) by (4.37), we obtain

$$\begin{aligned}
\frac{\frac{dx}{dt}}{\frac{dz}{dt}} &= \frac{-\kappa xy}{ly}, \\
\frac{dx}{dz} &= \frac{-\kappa}{l}x \text{ (simplify)}, \\
\frac{dx}{x} &= \frac{-\kappa}{l}dz \\
&\quad \text{(divide both sides by } x \text{ and multiply by } dz), \\
\int_0^t \frac{1}{x}dx &= \int_0^t \frac{-\kappa}{l}dz \text{ (integrate both sides from 0 to } t), \\
\ln(x(t)) - \ln(x(0)) &= -\frac{\kappa}{l}(z(t) - z(0)) \text{ (using integration rules)}, \\
\ln(x(t)) - \ln(x(0)) &= \frac{\kappa}{l}(z(0) - z(t)) \\
&\quad \text{(eliminate minus sign by taking negative of RHS)}, \\
\frac{x(t)}{x(0)} &= \exp\left(\frac{\kappa}{l}(z(0) - z(t))\right) \text{ (exponentiate both sides)}, \\
x(t) &= x(0)\exp\left(-\frac{\kappa}{l}(z(t))\right) \text{ (multiply with } x(0); z(0) \text{ is zero–} \\
&\quad \text{no recovered at time 0).}
\end{aligned} \tag{4.39, 4.40}$$

This expression for $x(t)$ now can be plugged into Eq. (4.38) which becomes

$$\frac{dz}{dt} = l\left(N - x_0\exp\left(-\frac{\kappa}{l}z\right) - z\right) \tag{4.41}$$

where $x(0)$ is written as x_0. Eq. (4.41) cannot be directly solved for z, but Kermack & McKendrick apply a useful trick: They expand the expression $\exp(-\frac{\kappa}{l}z)$ as exponential series (see Chap. 3), using only the first two terms, i.e.

$$\begin{aligned}
\exp\left(-\frac{\kappa}{l}z\right) &= \sum_{k=0}^{\infty}\frac{\left(-\frac{\kappa}{l}z\right)^k}{k!} \\
&\approx \frac{\left(-\frac{\kappa}{l}z\right)^0}{0!}+\frac{\left(-\frac{\kappa}{l}z\right)^1}{1!}+\frac{\left(-\frac{\kappa}{l}z\right)^2}{2!}, \\
\exp\left(-\frac{\kappa}{l}z\right) &\approx \frac{\kappa^2z^2}{l^2}-1-\frac{\kappa}{2l}z. \qquad (4.42)
\end{aligned}$$

Plugging the approximate expression (4.42) for $\exp(-\frac{\kappa}{l}z)$ into Eq. (4.41) the following results:

$$\begin{aligned}
\frac{dz}{dt} &= l\left(N-x_0\exp\left(-\frac{\kappa}{l}z\right)-z\right) \\
&= l\left(N-x_0\left(\frac{\kappa^2z^2}{l^2}-1-\frac{\kappa}{l}z\right)-z\right) \\
&= l\left(N-x_0+\left(\frac{\kappa}{l}x_0-1\right)z-\frac{x_0\kappa^2z^2}{2l^2}\right) \text{ (rearrange).} \qquad (4.43)
\end{aligned}$$

Remember that this is an approximation to $\frac{dz}{dt}$; the big advantage of this operation is the solvability of this system which is a Riccati equation.[4] The solution is quite "messy" (see Eq. (30) on p. 713):

$$z=\frac{l^2}{\kappa^2x_0}\left(\frac{\kappa}{l}x_0-1+Q\tanh\left(\frac{Q}{2}lt-\phi\right)\right) \qquad (4.44)$$

where $Q=\sqrt{(\frac{\kappa}{l}x_0-1)^2+2x_0y_0\frac{\kappa^2}{l^2}}$ and $\phi=\tanh^{-1}\left(\frac{\frac{\kappa}{l}x_0-1}{Q}\right)$. tanh is the *hyperbolic tangent* and $\tanh^{-1}$ is its inverse. This solution, which is an approximate one (because only the first two terms of the exponential series expansion were used) expresses $z(t)$, the cumulative number of "removals" by time t as a function of the infection and removal parameters, the initial numbers of susceptibles and infecteds, x_0 and y_0, and the time t.

The first derivative of that function, $\frac{dz}{dt}$, is the rate of increase (z can only increase) in the numbers removed; Kermack & McKendrick ingeniously fit this function to data on the weekly numbers of plague deaths on the island of Bombay in the early 20th century. Because of the high case fatality of plague at that time, the number of deaths is a good approximation to the number of removed. Even though details regarding the fitting process are omitted, the fit is visually remarkable (figure on p. 714). They also discuss the limitation of applying this model to plague (top of p. 715).

Now assume that the initial number of infecteds, y_0, is "neglected" such that x_0 is "almost" N, and z does not change over time, i.e. $\frac{dz}{dt}=0$; given that there was an outbreak, this can only be the case at the very end of the epidemic. Strictly, this will

[4] I owe this insight to the discussion of the Kermack & McKendrick paper in [1].

be at time ∞, but this is of no matter. Eq. (4.43) will then become:

$$\begin{aligned}
\frac{dz}{dt} &= l\left(N - x_0 + \left(\frac{\kappa}{l}x_0 - 1\right)z - \frac{x_0\kappa^2 z^2}{2l^2}\right), \\
0 &\approx l\left(N - N + \left(\frac{\kappa}{l}N - 1\right)z - \frac{N\kappa^2 z^2}{2l^2}\right) \qquad (4.45) \\
& \quad \text{(replacing } x_0 \text{ with } N \text{ and setting } \frac{dz}{dt} = 0\text{)}, \\
0 &\approx \left(\frac{\kappa}{l}N - 1\right) - \frac{N\kappa^2 z}{2l^2} \text{ (dividing by } l \text{ and } z\text{)}, \\
\frac{N\kappa^2 z}{2l^2} &\approx \left(\frac{\kappa}{l}N - 1\right) \text{ (adding } \frac{N\kappa^2 z}{2l^2} \text{ to both sides)}, \\
z &\approx \frac{2l^2}{\kappa^2 N}\left(\frac{\kappa}{l}N - 1\right) \text{ (manipulating to isolate } z \text{ on the left)}, \\
z &= \frac{2l}{\kappa N}\left(N - \frac{l}{\kappa}\right) \text{ (simplifying)}. \qquad (4.46)
\end{aligned}$$

Note that in Eq. (4.46) I have, somewhat "illegally", but to be consistent with Kermack & McKendrick, replaced the approximation sign ($\approx$) with an equal sign ($=$) and have put x_0 to N, which differs from Eq. (32) in the paper. This equation is very important, as it quantifies the ultimate size of the epidemic, even though it is based on various approximations.

Kermack & McKendrick state, regarding the trick to let y_0 disappear and set x_0 to N:

> *"This is obviously no limitation as y_0 the initial number of infected cases is usually small as compared with x_0." (p. 715, after Eq. (32))*

Question 4.q

Using the transmission model you developed (or I provided) for Question 4.q to verify the final size equation (4.46) quantitatively.

The statement:

> *"It is clear that when x_0, which is identical with N if y_0 be neglected, is equal to $\frac{l}{\kappa}$, no epidemic can take place." (p. 715, middle paragraph)*

This phrase, which may appear as modest, is often referred to as the *threshold theorem* and is one of the most important insights from this paper. It is based on the fact that an outbreak is only possible if $N > \frac{l}{\kappa}$.

A problem with Eq. (4.46) is the fact that, if $N < \frac{l}{\kappa}$, z becomes *negative*–z, however, must be *positive* ($z \geq 0$). I will ignore this difficulty, at least for now.

According to the threshold theorem, $\frac{l}{\kappa}$ is the threshold value for N. If N is just slightly above that value, say

$$N = \frac{l}{\kappa} + n, \qquad (4.47)$$

the size of the epidemic will be

$$\begin{aligned} z &= \frac{2l}{\kappa N}\left(N - \frac{l}{\kappa}\right) \\ &= \frac{2l}{\kappa N}\left(\left(\frac{l}{\kappa} + n\right) - \frac{l}{\kappa}\right) \text{ (substituting } \frac{l}{\kappa} + n \text{ for } N \text{ on right)} \\ &= 2\frac{l}{\kappa}\frac{n}{N} \text{ (simplifying)} \qquad (4.48) \\ &= 2(N-n)\frac{n}{N} \text{ (substituting } \frac{l}{\kappa} \text{ for } N-n\text{; see (4.47))} \\ &= 2n - \frac{2n^2}{N} \text{ (simplifying).} \qquad (4.49) \end{aligned}$$

Eq. (4.47), the (approximate) final size of a "small" epidemic, therefore is, as Kermack & McKendrick comment, "to a first approximation, equal to $2n$" (p. 715). This is justified by the fact that, n is very small, and N is very large.

Trying this out numerically, for example, using the model developed in answering Question 4.p, we see that this approximation is very inaccurate: Using the parameter values from the answer to Question 4.o ($\kappa = 0.00005$, $l = 0.25$), we calculate a threshold number of susceptibles as $\frac{l}{\kappa} = \frac{0.25}{0.00005} = 5{,}000$. So if we start out with, say, 5,001 susceptibles, such that $n = 1$, we would expect an epidemic to terminate with $z(\infty) \approx 2n = 2$. However, if we run this epidemic, with parameters used before and with a starting population of susceptibles of 5,001, the epidemic terminates with $z(\infty) \approx 99$. In the next section (11), Kermack & McKendrick generalize these results to non-constant rates, but I leave it to the reader to examine this.

4.3.2 (12): Extension to vector-borne diseases

Vector-borne diseases are diseases caused by viruses (e.g. yellow fever), bacteria (e.g. plague), protozoa (e.g. malaria), or nematodes (e.g. onchocerciasis) that are transmitted from one vertebrate host to the next by insects, such as mosquitoes, or arachnids, such as ticks. Typically, especially in the case of the protozoan or nematodal diseases, transmission is not "mechanical", such as by contaminated mouth parts, but requires completion of part of the parasites life cycle in the arthropod. Vector-borne diseases are of tremendous public health importance. Kermack & McKendrick did not see a fundamental reason against transferring their models of transmission to vector-borne diseases stating that

> *"It is not difficult to extend these results to such diseases as malaria or plague, in which transmission is through an intermediate host." (p. 718)*

They adapt Eq. (4.26) to reflect the two components of the transmission cycle, mosquito to human and human to mosquito:

$$-\frac{d\ln(x(t))}{dt} = \int_0^t \mathrm{A}'(\theta)v'(t-\theta)d\theta + \mathrm{A}'(t)y'(0) \qquad (4.50)$$

and

$$-\frac{d\ln(x'(t))}{dt} = \int_0^t \mathrm{A}(\theta)v(t-\theta)d\theta + \mathrm{A}(t)y(0) \tag{4.51}$$

where the *prime* (′) represents the quantities in the vector. Note that the typesetter seems to have omitted the minus sign on the left-hand side of the equations. The expressions corresponding to Eq. (4.33) are obtained from (4.50) and (4.51):

$$-\ln\left(\frac{1-p}{1-\frac{y(0)}{N}}\right) = \mathrm{A}'N'p', \tag{4.52}$$

$$-\ln\left(\frac{1-p'}{1-\frac{y'(0)}{N'}}\right) = \mathrm{A}Np. \tag{4.53}$$

As before, Kermack & McKendrick "neglect" $\frac{y'(0)}{N'}$ and $\frac{y(0)}{N}$, i.e. set these expressions to zero; this is justified by the fact that the starting number of infecteds is assumed to be small relative to the population. This results in expressions

$$-\ln(1-p) = \mathrm{A}'N'p', \tag{4.54}$$

$$-\ln(1-p') = \mathrm{A}Np. \tag{4.55}$$

Again, the natural logarithm in these two expressions is replaced with a partial logarithmic series, i.e. an approximation. The following property is used:

$\ln a = (a-1) - \frac{1}{2}(a-1)^2 + \frac{1}{3}(a-1)^3 - \frac{1}{4}(a-1)^4 + \cdots$, for $2 \geq a > 0$.
Let $a = 1-p$ and $(a-1) = -p$. Then, this series becomes

$$\ln(1-p) = -p - \frac{p^2}{2} - \frac{p^3}{3} - \frac{p^4}{4} - \cdots,$$

$$-\ln(1-p) = p + \frac{p^2}{2} + \frac{p^3}{3} + \frac{p^4}{4} + \cdots \text{ (multiplying by } -1\text{)},$$

$$-\ln(1-p) \approx p + \frac{p^2}{2} \text{ (ignoring powers of } p \text{ of 3 and higher)}. \tag{4.56}$$

Using this relationship, Eqs. (4.54) and (4.55) become

$$p + \frac{p^2}{2} \approx \mathrm{A}'N'p', \tag{4.57}$$

$$p' + \frac{p'^2}{2} \approx \mathrm{A}Np. \tag{4.58}$$

Multiplying the two equations–left-hand side of (4.57) with left-hand side of (4.58) and doing the same for the right-hand sides–the following results:

$$\begin{aligned}
\left(p+\frac{p^2}{2}\right)\left(p'+\frac{p'^2}{2}\right) &\approx (\mathrm{A}'N'p')(\mathrm{A}Np),\\
p\left(1+\frac{p}{2}\right)p'\left(1+\frac{p'}{2}\right) &\approx (\mathrm{A}'\mathrm{A}NN'pp')\\
&\quad \text{(factoring } p,\, p' \text{ left and rearranging right)},\\
\left(1+\frac{p}{2}\right)\left(1+\frac{p'}{2}\right) &\approx \mathrm{A}'\mathrm{A}NN' \text{ (dividing both sides by } pp'),\\
1+\frac{p}{2}+\frac{p'}{2}+\frac{pp'}{4} &\approx \mathrm{A}'\mathrm{A}NN' \text{ (multiplying out parentheses)},\\
\frac{p}{2}+\frac{p'}{2} &\approx \mathrm{A}'\mathrm{A}NN' - 1 \qquad (4.59)\\
&\quad \text{(“ignoring” product } \frac{pp'}{4} \text{ an subtracting 1}\\
&\quad \text{from both sides).}
\end{aligned}$$

Note that Kermack & McKendrick use an equal sign (=) instead of the approximation sign (≈).

As p and p' represent the fractions of humans and vector arthropods eventually becoming infected, they must be non-negative. Therefore, considering expression (4.59), $\mathrm{A}'\mathrm{A}NN'$ must be larger than 1 for a true epidemic to occur; it cannot be smaller than 1, as $\frac{p}{2}+\frac{p'}{2}$ would be negative and can only be 1 when both p and p' are zero.

If we let $\mathrm{A}'\mathrm{A}NN' = 1$, it becomes clear that there is no unique threshold value for humans or vector arthropods, but that there is a threshold *product* NN'. If we set $N' = N_0'$ and let the corresponding threshold value for N be N_0 (such that NN_0' is the threshold product) we can solve this equation for N_0 to get $N_0 = \frac{1}{\mathrm{A}'\mathrm{A}N_0'}$. If N exceeds N_0 only by a little bit (n), we can write $N = N_0 + n = \frac{1}{\mathrm{A}'\mathrm{A}N_0'} + n$. Further, again “ignoring” powers of p of 2 and higher (because those terms become small), we can solve expression (4.57) for p' and get $p' = \frac{p}{\mathrm{A}'N'}$. Then, we substitute these values for N, N' and p' into expression (4.59) to obtain

$$\begin{aligned}
\frac{p}{2}+\frac{p'}{2} &= \mathrm{A}'\mathrm{A}NN' - 1,\\
\frac{p}{2}+\frac{p}{2\mathrm{A}'N'} &= \mathrm{A}'\mathrm{A}N_0' \times \left(\frac{1}{\mathrm{A}'\mathrm{A}N_0'} + n\right) - 1,\\
p\left(1+\frac{1}{\mathrm{A}'N'}\right) &= 2\mathrm{A}'\mathrm{A}N_0' \times \left(\frac{1}{\mathrm{A}'\mathrm{A}N_0'} + n\right) - 2\\
&\quad \text{(substituting for } p' \text{ and multiplying by 2)},\\
p\left(\frac{\mathrm{A}'N'+1}{\mathrm{A}'N'}\right) &= 2\frac{\mathrm{A}'\mathrm{A}N_0'}{\mathrm{A}'\mathrm{A}N_0'} + 2n\mathrm{A}'\mathrm{A}N_0' - 2\\
&\quad \text{(manipulating and multiplying out RHS)},\\
p &= \frac{2+2n\mathrm{A}'\mathrm{A}N_0' - 2}{\mathrm{A}'N'+1}\mathrm{A}'N' \text{ (manipulating some more)},
\end{aligned}$$

$$p = \frac{2n}{N_0}\frac{A'N'}{A'N'+1} \tag{4.60}$$

(making use of $A'AN_0' = \frac{1}{N_0}$ and manipulating some more).

On the last page of the paper (pp. 719–720), Kermack & McKendrick derive a result analogous to (4.48), and I leave this up to the reader to explore (this should pose no major hurdles). Instead, I will finish this chapter with a question.

Question 4.r

The following chapter is entirely devoted to mathematical models of vector-borne (i.e. mosquito-borne) disease transmission. As preparation, consider the exploration of Kermack & McKendrick of that territory by generalizing their modeling approach to the vector-borne situation. Is there anything that strikes you as particularly problematic?

Appendix 4.A

Kermack & McKendrick's conclusion that there was no explicit solution to (4.25) is followed by the following statement:

> *"It may, however, be pointed out that this is an integral equation similar to Volterra's equation:*
>
> $$f(t) = \phi(t) + \int_0^t \mathrm{N}(t,\theta)\phi(\theta)d\theta$$
>
> *except that in place of $f(t)$ we have $\frac{d\log f(t)}{dt}$." (p. 705, following quote on page 68)*

Usually, the *Volterra integral equation of the second kind*, like the one in the quote is displayed as

$$\phi(t) = f(t) + \int_0^t \mathrm{N}(t,\theta)\phi(\theta)d\theta.$$

This equation is a special case of a *Fredholm integral equation of the second kind*

$$\phi(t) = f(t) + \lambda\int_a^b \mathrm{N}(t,\theta)\phi(\theta)d\theta$$

which can be solved iteratively (see top expression on p. 706) as

$$x(t) = f_0(t) + \lambda f_1(t) + \lambda^2 f_2(t) + \cdots.$$

This method, however, is rooted in the Fredholm equation above. Here, however, we have $\frac{d\log\phi(t)}{dt}$ instead of $\phi(t)$. This, in my opinion, precludes this recursive solution.

Appendix 4.B Answers

4.a This question is so open-ended that it almost merits its own book. What I was thinking of is the works of Hamer and Soper which we discussed in the previous chapter. The important point is the insight that epidemic dynamics do not require changes in biological characteristics of the infectious agent or in the transmission process. Importantly, the ceasing of an epidemic is not necessarily–and not usually–caused by the absolute exhaustion of the susceptibles.

4.b Because ψ is a *real* number as opposed to an integer $v_{1,1}$ and therefore, generally, $v_{t,\theta}$ must be real numbers, too. Therefore, $v_{t,\theta}$ cannot truly represent the numbers of infectious in that class (indexed by time t and time since infection, θ) such as one, two, three, etc. It therefore truly represents a *quantity* rather than a *number of subjects* with certain characteristics. As we will see, this is a fundamental characteristic of difference equation or differential equation models.

4.c $\psi_\theta v_{t,\theta} = v_{t,\theta} - v_{t+1,\theta+1}$ is true because the number of infecteds (once they have been infected) is *via* the removal process which is determined by the parameter ψ_θ which is the proportion infected who are removed during interval θ (in terms of time since infection). The change in the number of subjects who were infected at time $t-\theta$ from the current (t) to the next ($t+1$) time interval must therefore be the current number ($v_{t,\theta}$) times the removal proportion ψ_θ. That change is $v_{t,\theta} - v_{t+1,\theta+1}$ the order of which, at first glance, may seem confusing. But from what has been said, $v_{t,\theta} > v_{t+1,\theta+1}$.

4.d An appropriate term for $\mathbf{B}_\theta$ would in that case (θ the probability of dying rather than removal) be *survival.*

4.e The one truly fundamental assumption here is that infection does not arise *de novo*, but, rather, depends on some kind of contact with an infectious individual. The type of contact varies by infectious agent studied: For a sexually transmitted agent the nature of that contact is clearly different from the contact required for the infection of a respiratory virus. In some instances, of course, infection can occur *via* fomites which are objects that have been contaminated with the infectious agent.

4.f The expression $v_t = x(t)\sum_1^t \phi_\theta v_{t,\theta}$ describes the number of new infections given the number of those still susceptible ($x(t)$) and given all infectious "individuals". As pointed out in Question 4.a, the numbers $v_{t,\theta}$ do not truly represent individuals, as a fraction ψ_θ recovers at the end of "infection age" θ.
If $x(t)$ is assumed to be one, i.e. $x(t) \equiv 1$, then (if $t > 3$)

$$\begin{aligned} v_t &= \sum_1^t \phi_\theta v_{t,\theta} \\ &= \phi_1 v_{t,1} + \phi_2 v_{t,2} + \cdots + \phi_t v_{t,t}. \end{aligned}$$

Therefore, $\phi_\theta v_{t,\theta}$ represents the number (again, not an integer, but a positive real number) of new infections resulting from $v_{t,\theta}$ infectious individuals *per susceptible*

individual and therefore ϕ_θ is the number of new infections generated *per [one] infectious individual per susceptible individual.*
Kermack & McKendrick write that this "follows since the chance of an infection is proportional to the number of infected on the one hand, and to the number not yet infected on the other" (p. 703, lower half). This, actually, is a discrete-time variant of the "mass action" principle we have encountered in [8].

4.g Applying the general definition of $v_t = v_{t,0}$ to expression $x(t) = N - \sum_0^t v_{t,0} = N - v_{0,0} - v_{1,0} - \ldots - v_{t,0}$ (first line of expression (3)) we get $x(t) = N - v_{0,0} - v_{1,0} - \ldots - v_{t,0} = N - \sum_0^t v_t$. However, for $t = 0$ $v_t = v_0 = v_{0,0} + y_0$ (see paragraph "New infections") which can be solved for $v_{0,0} = v_0 - y_0$. Therefore, $v_{0,0}$ has to be replaced by $v_0 - y_0$ and we can write the expression as $x(t) = N - v_{0,0} - v_{1,0} - \ldots - v_{t,0} = N - v_0 - y_0 - v_1 - \ldots - v_t = N - \sum_0^t v_t - y_0$. This is the expression given by Kermack & McKendrick.

4.h B_θ represents the "proportion" surviving (i.e. not being removed from infection by either death or recovery) through interval θ. Note that here time interval refers to the time since infection. This can be written as $\mathrm{B}_\theta = \prod_{i=0}^{\theta-1}(1 - \psi_i)$. Note that this is the product of the survival proportions for each post-infection interval up to $\psi_{\theta-1}$. In a probabilistic interpretation, therefore, ψ_n corresponds to an interval survival probability. If we let R be a random variable that represents the time interval during which recovery (or death) occurs, then $\mathrm{B}_\theta = \Pr(R > \theta)$, i.e. the probability to survive to time interval θ (not die before θ). Note that this probability is equivalent to the probability to survive the first interval $(1 - \psi_0)$, then survive the next interval $(1 - \psi_1)$, etc., i.e. $(1 - \psi_0) \times (1 - \psi_1) \times \cdots \times (1 - \psi_{\theta-1})$–this is the definition of B (see expression (4.1)).
C_θ is the proportion of those being removed at the end of interval $\theta + 1$. To be removed after that interval, an individual needs to survive up to that interval. The corresponding probability therefore can be interpreted as a conditional probability, $\Pr(R = \theta + 1 | R > \theta)$.[5]
For A_θ, finally, we first have to consider the meaning of ϕ_θ, the "rate of infectivity at age θ". It really is the "quantity" of new infections *one* infectious individual, having been infected for θ intervals, causes in *one* susceptible in one time interval. To quantify the number of new infections in an interval caused by individuals of given "age" ϕ_θ therefore has to be multiplied by both the number of such individuals and the number of susceptible individuals (see expression (4.2)). As this is not bound to be between 0 and 1, i.e. can be larger than 1, it cannot be a probability, and A_θ cannot therefore be expressed as a probability.
A final note regarding the "interval survival" probability (i.e. the probability of not recovering during a given interval, given infectivity at the beginning of the interval). This will be of importance later. The recovery process in interval θ is driven by a recovery rate, say λ_θ. The probability ψ_θ (not to recover in interval θ) can then be

[5] The notation $A|B$ indicates a conditional event "A given B".

written as $\psi_\theta = \exp(-\lambda_\theta t_\theta)$ where t_θ is the duration of interval θ. The reason for this is as follows: If λ_θ is a rate that drives a *Poisson process* in which the expected number of events per time unit is λ_θ then the time t between two adjacent events follows an exponential distribution:

$$f(t|\lambda_\theta) = \lambda_\theta \exp(-\lambda_\theta t).$$

Furthermore, the probability that t is larger than t_θ is

$$F(t_\theta|\lambda_\theta) = \exp(-\lambda_\theta t_\theta);$$

$F(\cdot|\lambda_\theta)$ denotes the cumulative distribution function of $f(\cdot|\lambda_\theta)$, and this is ψ_θ, accordingly! The one little problem with this analogy is this. We are not operating in a *stochastic* context here, but in a *deterministic* one; talking about probabilities therefore is not quite adequate–we will get back to this later.

4.i This is a continuation of the rambling answer to Question 4.g. Let us consider the most basic of the three parameters, B_θ (this parameter is a product of the $\prod_{t=0}^{\theta}(1-\psi_t) = (1-\psi_0)(1-\psi_1) \times \cdots \times (1-\psi_\theta)$). Following the argument in the answer to Question 4.g, we can therefore write:

$$\begin{aligned}
B_\theta &= \prod_{t=0}^{\theta}(1-\psi_t) \\
&= \prod_{t=0}^{\theta}\exp(-\lambda_t) \\
&= \exp\left(-\sum_{t=0}^{\theta}\lambda_t\right) \text{ (property of exponents, } \prod_i \exp(x_i) = \exp(\sum_i x_i)).
\end{aligned}$$

This assumes that the rates of each interval refer to the expected number of events per interval (otherwise, the rates would have to be multiplied by the interval length). If we let the time intervals become infinitesimally small, the sums become integrals again and $B_\theta = \exp(-\int_{t=0}^{\theta}\lambda_t dt)$. Note that this corresponds to the survival function which is the probability to survive to time t if the driving rate, λ_t, is *memoryless*. The memoryless property refers to the independence of events or, more specifically, the independence of event-to-event times: The time to the next event cannot be predicted from the time to the previous event. Now we make use of an important property of exponents to the base e (also see Chap. 3, p. 41):

$$\lim_{a \to 0} \frac{\exp(a)}{1+a} = 1. \tag{4.60}$$

This implies that, if a is "small", $\exp(a) \sim 1+a$, or, what is more relevant to this discussion,

$$\begin{aligned}
\exp(-a) &\sim 1+(-a) = 1-a \text{ (using (4.60))}, \\
-\exp(-a) &\sim -1+a \text{ (multiplying both sides by } -1), \\
1-\exp(-a) &\sim a \text{ (adding 1 to both sides).}
\end{aligned} \tag{4.61}$$

"Small" ψ_t, therefore, can in approximation be substituted by $1 - \exp(-\psi_t)$. So if B_θ is defined in terms of interval recovery probabilities (or proportions) $1 - \psi_t$ then, again only if ψ_t is small, it is appropriate to state:

$$\begin{aligned} B_\theta &\sim \exp\left(-\sum_{t=0}^{\theta}\psi_t\right) \\ &\sim \exp\left(-\int_{t=0}^{\theta}\psi_t dt\right) \text{ (if the length of the time intervals approaches 0),} \end{aligned}$$

but the $\sim$ cannot be replaced by $=$. Accordingly, $\psi_t \neq \lambda_t$. However, for better consistency, we will be using ψ_t where λ_t should be used.
From here, the other parameters follow much more easily:

- $C_\theta = \psi_\theta B_\theta = \psi_\theta \exp\left(-\int_{t=0}^{\theta}\psi_t dt\right)$. This is a failure time distribution for time-varying failure rates, i.e. a probability density function: C_θ represents the probability density for failure "time" θ (remember that θ does not correspond to *time*, but to *time since infection*). Again, the lines between a stochastic and a deterministic approach are blurred.
- $A_\theta = \phi_\theta B_\theta = \phi_\theta \exp\left(-\int_{t=0}^{\theta}\psi_t dt\right)$. The parameter A_θ does not have an interpretation as a probability density or survival probability; it is, however, the infection pressure exerted by one individual at time θ, weighted by the probability not to recover before θ. In fact, $\int_{t=0}^{\theta} A_\theta dt = E_t(\phi_t)$, i.e. the expected or *average infection pressure*, while $\int_{t=0}^{\theta}\phi_\theta dt$ is the *total infection pressure* exerted by an infectious individual.

4.j An intuitive argument would go as follows: The two expressions,

$$\int_0^t A(\theta)v(t-\theta)d\theta$$

and

$$\int_0^t A(t-\theta)v(\theta)d\theta,$$

are very similar; only for the first one, if we set $\theta = 0$, the kernel $(A(\theta)v(t-\theta))$ is $A(0)v(t)$, and if we set $\theta = t$, it becomes $A(t)v(0)$. For the second expression it is just the opposite. So the functions seem the same, but the "direction of integration" with respect to θ is just reverse ("left-to-right" vs. "right-to-left"). The result should be the same, as the area under the curve should remain unchanged.
The expression $\int_0^t A(\theta)v(t-\theta)d\theta$ is referred to as a *convolution integral*. A property of the convolution integral $\int_0^t f(x)v(t-x)dx$ is

$$\int_0^t f(x)v(t-x)dx = \int_0^t f(t-x)v(t)dx$$

which justifies the "exchange of arguments".

The following argument can be made without using convolution integrals. Let $f(\theta) = \mathrm{A}(\theta)v(t-\theta)$ (from Eq. (4.19)). Then we can write

$$\int_0^t \mathrm{A}(\theta)v(t-\theta)d\theta = \int_0^t f(\theta)d\theta.$$

Define $\theta^* = t-\theta$. It follows that $f(\theta^*) = \mathrm{A}(t-\theta)v(\theta)$ (from Eq. (4.20))–this can be seen by plugging the definition of θ^* into the expression for $f(\cdot)$:

$$\begin{aligned} f(\theta^*) &= \mathrm{A}(\theta^*)v(t-\theta^*) \\ &= \mathrm{A}(t-\theta)v(t-(t-\theta)) \text{ (plugging-in } 1-\theta \text{ for } \theta^*) \\ &= \mathrm{A}(t-\theta)v(\theta). \end{aligned}$$

The final expression is from $\int_0^t \mathrm{A}(t-\theta)v(\theta)d\theta$ in Eq. (4.20) which also could be written as $\int_0^t f(\theta^a st)d\theta$. Following the argument from the answer to Question 4.k (see below), we write

$$\begin{aligned} \int_{\theta^*=0}^{t} f(\theta^*)d\theta^* &= \int_{\theta=t}^{0} f(\theta^*)d\theta^* \\ &\quad \text{(new limits of integration by expression } \theta^* \text{ in terms of } \theta; \\ &\quad \text{that } \theta = t \text{ is equivalent to } \theta^* = 0) \\ &= -\int_{\theta=t}^{0} f(\theta^*)d\theta \\ &\quad \text{(because } \theta^* = t-\theta\text{—see the answer to Question 4.k)} \\ &= \int_{\theta=0}^{t} f(\theta^*)d\theta \\ &\quad \text{(The elimination of the "}-\text{" sign results in reversion} \\ &\quad \text{of limits).} \end{aligned}$$

In summary, $\int_{\theta^*=0}^{t} f(\theta^*)d\theta^* = \int_{\theta=0}^{t} f(\theta^*)d\theta$ or, plugging-in the expressions for $f(\cdot)$, i.e. $f(\theta^*) = \mathrm{A}(t-\theta)v(\theta)$ and $f(\theta) = \mathrm{A}(\theta)v(t\theta)$, respectively,

$$\int_0^t \mathrm{A}(\theta)v(t-\theta)d\theta = \int_0^t \mathrm{A}(t-\theta)v(\theta)d\theta$$

which is what we wanted to verify.

4.k First consider the equation

$$\frac{d\mathrm{A}_{t-\theta}}{d(t-\theta)} = -\frac{d\mathrm{A}_{t-\theta}}{d\theta}$$

and remember the chain rule of derivation,

$$\frac{dz}{dx} = \frac{dz}{dy}\frac{dy}{dx},$$

where $y = f(x)$ is a function of x and $z = g(f(x)) = g(x)$ is a function of y. So the left-hand side of the expression above could be written as

$$\frac{d\mathrm{A}_{t-\theta}}{d(t-\theta)}\frac{d(t-\theta)}{d(t-\theta)}$$

(multiplying by $\frac{d(t-\theta)}{d(t-\theta)}$ is multiplying by 1) and the right-hand side can be written as

$$\frac{d\mathrm{A}_{t-\theta}}{d(t-\theta)}\frac{d(t-\theta)}{d(\theta)}.$$

The only difference between the two is the last denominator. In fact, $\frac{d(t-\theta)}{d(t-\theta)} = 1$, but $\frac{d(t-\theta)}{d(\theta)} = -1$. The first is true because $\frac{dx}{dx} = 1$; the second holds because $\frac{d(-x)}{dx} = -1$; note that the t in the expression is inconsequential because its derivative with respect to x is zero.

4.l This answer almost exactly mirrors the answer to Question 4.j. The most straightforward answer uses the property of convolution integrals (see the answer to Question 4.j).

4.m If time is discrete, the left-hand side of the equation

$$\int_0^\infty \int_0^t \mathrm{A}(\theta)v(t-\theta)d\theta dt = \int_0^\infty \int_0^t \mathrm{A}(\theta)v(t-\theta)d\theta dt$$

becomes

$$\sum_{t=0}^{\infty}\left(\sum_{\theta=0}^{t}\mathrm{A}(\theta)v(t-\theta)\Delta\theta\right)\Delta t.$$

This double sum is computed by starting with the starting value for $t = 0$ for the outer sum and using that for the inner sum which will have a starting value of 0 and an end value of 0. So the first element of the sum is:

$$\begin{aligned}
&\text{For } t=0, \sum_{\theta=0}^{0}\mathrm{A}(\theta)v(t-\theta)\Delta\theta: && \mathrm{A}(0)v(0)\Delta\theta\,\Delta t\\
&\text{For } t=1, \sum_{\theta=0}^{1}\mathrm{A}(\theta)v(t-\theta)\Delta\theta: &+& \mathrm{A}(0)v(1)\Delta\theta\,\Delta t + \mathrm{A}(1)v(0)\Delta\theta\,\Delta t\\
&\text{For } t=2, \sum_{\theta=0}^{2}\mathrm{A}(\theta)v(t-\theta)\Delta\theta: &+& \mathrm{A}(0)v(2)\Delta\theta\,\Delta t + \mathrm{A}(1)v(1)\Delta\theta\,\Delta t\\
&&& + \mathrm{A}(2)v(0)\Delta\theta\,\Delta t\\
&\text{etc.}
\end{aligned}$$

These terms can be rearranged in the following way:

$$\begin{aligned}
&(\mathrm{A}(0)+\mathrm{A}(1)+\mathrm{A}(2)+\cdots)\,\Delta\theta\,(v(0)+v(1)+v(2)+\cdots)\,\Delta t\\
&= \sum_{\theta=0}^{\infty}\mathrm{A}(\theta)\Delta\theta\sum_{\theta=0}^{\infty}v(t)\Delta t.
\end{aligned}$$

If we let the "time steps" $\Delta\theta$ and Δt become infinitesimally small, we obtain the expression we were looking for, i.e.

$$\lim_{\Delta\theta,\Delta t\to 0}\sum_{\theta=0}^{\infty}\mathrm{A}(\theta)\Delta\theta\sum_{t=0}^{\infty}v(t)\Delta t=\left(\int_{\theta=0}^{\infty}\mathrm{A}(\theta)d\theta\right)\times\left(\int_{t=0}^{\infty}v(t)dt\right).$$

4.n Eq. (4.17) can, as Kermack & McKendrick state, be treated "in a similar manner" Eq. (4.14) was treated. Most importantly, by integrating both sides with respect to t, we obtain

$$\begin{aligned}\int_0^{\infty}y(t)dt &= \int_0^{\infty}\int_0^{t}\mathrm{B}(\theta)v(t-\theta)d\theta+\mathrm{B}(t)y(0)dt\\ &= \int_0^{\infty}\int_0^{t}\mathrm{B}(\theta)v(t-\theta)d\theta dt+\int_0^{\infty}\mathrm{B}(t)y(0)dt\\ &= \int_0^{t}v(t)dt\int_0^{\infty}\mathrm{B}(\theta)d\theta+\int_0^{\infty}\mathrm{B}(t)y(0)dt \text{ (See comment } *)\\ &= NP\int_0^{\infty}\mathrm{B}(\theta)d\theta+\int_0^{\infty}\mathrm{B}(t)y(0)dt \text{ (See comment } **).\end{aligned}$$

$*$ To get from $\int_0^t v(t)dt\int_0^{\infty}\mathrm{B}(\theta)d\theta$ to $\int_0^i nftyv(t)dt\int_0^{\infty}\mathrm{B}(\theta)d\theta$ I made use of the property of convolution integrals illustrated by Eq. (4.28).

$**$ $\int_0^t v(t)dt=Np$ because the integral represents the total number of infections in the epidemic, which is Np (remember that p is the proportion eventually infected).

4.o The removal parameter l is easier to interpret than κ: It is the daily rate of removal from the infected class. The reciprocal of l, $\frac{1}{l}$, is the "average" duration of infectiousness. The quotes are a reminder of the fact that this is a deterministic model, so averages do not apply. We can settle on a "reasonable" duration of infectiousness, e.g. 4 days. That would correspond to a rate of 0.25 per day. The correspondence of the duration and the rate is not really trivial, but can be intuitively understood as follows: In a stochastic framework, the time to removal t driven by a memory-less rate l (i.e. removal independent of duration of infectiousness) is distributed according to the exponential distribution: $f(t)l\exp(-lt)$. The mean/average time to recovery would be $\mu(t)=\frac{1}{l}$.
Let β be the number of secondary infections an index case generates in a single day in a wholly susceptible population (nobody is immune). Now, assume that only $x(t)$ individuals are susceptible at time t, out of the whole population of N individuals. As not every potentially infectious contact results in infection because of those who are already immune, the daily rate of new case generation is not β anymore, but $\beta\times\frac{x(t)}{N}$: The transmission rate is decreased proportionally to proportion of the population still susceptible. This expression can be rearranged to give

$$x(t)\frac{\beta}{N}.$$

If there is not just one infected but y infecteds, therefore, the daily rate of new infection generation is

$$x(t)y(t)\frac{\beta}{N}.$$

In Eqs. (4.35) and (4.36) we have $\mp xy\kappa$ instead. Therefore, $\kappa = \frac{\beta}{N}$, i.e. the transmission parameter κ is the *daily rate of case generation by one infected in a wholly susceptible population, divided by the population size N*. A starting point for the value could be the number of secondary cases resulting on average from one infection, given a totally susceptible population, say 2. If infectiousness lasts 4 days, the daily infection rate deriving from one infectious would be $\frac{2}{4} = 0.5 = \beta$. To obtain κ, that number has to be divided by the population size, say 10,000, which would give $\kappa = \frac{\beta}{10{,}000} = \frac{2}{4\times 10{,}000} = 0.00005$.

4.p Possibly the most difficult part of this question for many is to understand what is asked of them. While the differential equations describe the flow in and out of compartments (here x = susceptible, y = infectious, and z = removed), to really understand what is going on, we also have to know the numerical results. Our ease of access to numerical solutions of ordinary differential equations has rendered attempts to solve these equations of lesser concern. So what I was asking for are numerical solutions to these equations. Such numerical solutions can be obtained very easily today, with numerical algorithms implemented in many different software packages. The simplest algorithm, called Euler's method, naturally follows from discretizing the Kermack & McKendrick model. Starting with the initial conditions, the following steps are repeated:

1. Calculate Eqs. (4.35), (4.36), and (4.37) for current values of x, y, and z—remember, this is the "current rate of change" in the respective variable.
2. Multiply the resulting numbers (rate of change) with the duration of the time step, Δt—this represents the *amount of change.*
3. Add these amounts of change for x, y and z to the respective variables to get the new "current values".
4. Repeat until desired time is reached.

This model is implemented in R and MS Excel (online material). The performance, especially of Euler's method, increases with decreasing time step.

4.q First, plug-in parameter values into Eq. (4.46). Choosing the values I propose in the answer to Question 4.o (you can obviously choose your own values) with $\kappa = 0.00005$ and $l = 0.25$:

$$\begin{aligned} z &= \frac{2l}{x_0\kappa}\left(x_0 - \frac{l}{\kappa}\right) \\ &= \frac{2\times 0.25}{9{,}999\times 0.00005}\left(9{,}999 - \frac{0.25}{0.00005}\right) \\ &= 4{,}999.5. \end{aligned}$$

Using the same parameters and initial conditions in the model and letting it run until the epidemic is clearly over, we can look at the last value for z. For the Euler method model, the final size is 7969.85, while for the Runge–Kutta solution it is quite similar at 7968.46. But clearly, the difference with the analytic final size of almost 5,000 is big.

4.r This is, of course, a wide open question that can be answered in many different ways. One of the most obvious problems, however, may be the symmetric treatment of human (or, more generally, the *vertebrate*) host and the arthropod vector. The roles of these two necessary components of the transmission cycle, however, are far from symmetrical. One of the features that are particularly important to mosquito-borne transmission, owing to the generally short life span of these insects, is the crucial role of mosquito mortality (low probability of surviving the "extrinsic incubation period", until they are ready to transmit) and thus of vector demographics. Some of that can, of course, be accommodated by the parameter A'. Such a general treatment may not be adequate to capture essential features of vector-borne transmission.

Appendix 4.C Supplementary material

Supplementary material related to this chapter can be found online at http://dx.doi.org/10.1016/B978-0-12-802260-3.00004-3.

References

[1] Nicolas Bacaër, A Short History of Mathematical Population Dynamics, Springer Science & Business Media, 2011.
[2] Danile Bernoulli, Essai d'une nouvelle analyse de la mortalité causée par lat petite Vérole, & des avantages de l'inoculation pour la prévenir, 1760, pp. 1–45.
[3] V. Fock, Über eine Klasse von Integralgleichungen, Mathematische Zeitschrift 21 (1) (1924) 161–173.
[4] William Heaton Hamer, The Milroy Lectures on Epidemic Disease in England: The Evidence of Variability and of Persistency of Type, Bedford Press, 1906.
[5] M. Kermack, A.G. McKendrick, Contributions to the mathematical theory of epidemics. Part I, Proceedings of the Royal Society. Series A, Containing Papers of a Mathematical and Physical Character 115 (5) (1927) 700–721.
[6] Ronald Ross, An application of the theory of probabilities to the study of a priori pathometry. Part I, Proceedings of the Royal Society of London. Series A, Containing papers of a mathematical and physical character (1916) 204–230.
[7] Ronald Ross, Hilda P. Hudson, An application of the theory of probabilities to the study of a priori pathometry. Part II, Proceedings of the Royal Society of London A: Mathematical, Physical and Engineering Sciences 93 (650) (1917) 212–225, The Royal Society.
[8] H.E. Soper, The interpretation of periodicity in disease prevalence, Journal of the Royal Statistical Society (1929) 34–73.

R. Ross (1910, 1911) and G. Macdonald (1952) on the persistence of malaria

Contents

5.1 Introduction

This chapter mostly deals with two pieces of work that were separated by almost half a century. The first one is a book by Sir Ronald Ross [2] who received the *Nobel Prize in Physiology or Medicine* in 1902 for his work on the life cycle of the malaria parasite. Ross was a hugely and widely talented, but controversial, scientist, and the reader is referred to abundant published material casting a doubtful light on his personality. This aspect of Ross will, to stay consistent with my approach, be completely ignored. This book is an encyclopedic work on malaria, but I will discuss only a few pages that develop a quantitative framework for malaria transmission. Note that the Nobel Prize was awarded for his parasitological contributions, but he may have perceived mathematical epidemiology to be his true calling. This is complemented by a brief discussion of a short paper by Ross [3] that focused on some more developed mathematical aspects. Macdonald continued Ross's work, and his paper [1], which I will explore here, was published almost 50 years after Ross's book. His formulation of mosquito-borne transmission is sometimes referred to as the "Ross–Macdonald model".

A Historical Introduction to Mathematical Modeling of Infectious Diseases. DOI: 10.1016/B978-0-12-802260-3.00005-5

5.2 Ross: What keeps malaria going?

In Chap. V (Malaria in the community), on page 153 of his more than 600 pages long book [2], Ross sets out to develop his quantitative theory of malaria emergence and persistence. In Sect. 27 ("Conditions required for the Production of New Infections in a Locality"), he spells out the chain of events necessary for transmission of malaria in a specific location. These events can be paraphrased as follows:

1. A person with sufficient levels of malaria *gametocytes*, the form of the parasite which is infectious to mosquitoes, must be present.
2. A mosquito of a species that is *vector-competent*[1] for malaria must be present and must ingest a large enough amount of blood and thus of gametocytes. This will always be one of the genus *Anopheles*; the species depends on the malaria species; in the case of *Plasmodium falciparum*, the most dangerous form, the main vector mosquito species complex is *Anopheles gambiae*.
3. The mosquito must survive long enough to allow *sporozoites*, the form of the parasite infectious to humans, to develop.
4. Finally, that same mosquito must succeed in biting a susceptible human, thus completing the cycle. Actually, to fully complete the cycle, the new case or cases must have gametocytes that are infectious for mosquitoes in their blood.

He continues with the following question:

> *"Let us suppose that we have to do with a population of 1,000 people living over an area in which indigenous malaria does not exist; and suppose that one of these people is an imported case with suitable gametids in his blood. Next, suppose that a single suitable Anopheline is liberated within the area. What are the chances that this insect will ever cause a new infection?"*

So, clearly, he wants to approach the necessary chain of events numerically and lays down some "reasonable" assumptions regarding some of the parameters:

> *"[S]uppose that the chances are 4 to 1 against [a mosquito biting a human being]. Next, we observe that as there is only one infected person among the 1,000 people in the place, and as the particular Anopheline*[2] *liberated in the area may bite any one of these people, the chances are 1,000 to 1 against its happening to bite the patient, even if it succeeds in biting at all."* (p. 154)

[1] *Vector competence* refers to the ability of an insect (or other arthropod vector, such as a tick) to acquire infection from a vertebrate host and to transmit it back to another vertebrate host.

[2] Only mosquitoes of certain species of the genus *Anopheles* can transmit human malaria parasites, *Plasmodium falciparum, P. vivax, P. malariae, P. ovale*.

Question 5.a

According to Ross's statement, what is the probability of one mosquito (and we are *only* referring here to competent vectors of malaria, such as *An. gambiae*) biting the infectious human (i.e. one carrying gametocytes)?

In order to be able to transmit the malaria parasite to another human, the mosquito must survive long enough for the parasites to complete their life cycle and of sporozoites to form. This process requires about a week. As Ross comments, "not all mosquitoes live so long". Ross assumes a probability to survive from blood meal to infectiousness of $\frac{1}{3}$ and a probability of 0.25 that the now infectious mosquito succeeds to bite another human. Given these quantitative assumptions, the probability that one *vector-competent* mosquito, released into a population of 1,000 people with only *one* carrying gametocytes, would merely be $\frac{1}{48{,}000}$, which would make a secondary infection resulting from the index case exceedingly unlikely! Ross then continues with several more thought experiments and concludes that the risk of new malaria infections depends not only on the number of (vector-competent) mosquitoes, but also on the number of infectious people.

But finally, he ventures to introduce more formal definitions of parameters and variables (p. 155):

p is the number of size of the "local population".

m is the proportion of people with malaria; mp thus is the number of people with malaria.

i is the proportion of malaria infected people with *gametids* (Ross uses this term; today, this stage of *Plasmodia*, the form infectious to mosquitoes, is referred to as *gametocytes*).

a is the number of *Anopheline* mosquitoes of a species vector competent for malaria transmission per person, such that $a \times p$ is the total number of such mosquitoes.

b is the proportion of uninfected mosquitoes that succeed in biting a person, possibly acquiring malaria infection.

s is the proportion of mosquitoes which will live long enough to allow for the development of sporozoites (form of the malaria parasite which is infectious to humans).

b is the proportion of infectious mosquitoes biting a person (note this is the same as the proportion of uninfected mosquitoes biting a human).

The "number of Anophelines compared with the number of persons with gametids" thus is $aimp$, or more clearly stated, the numbers of mosquitoes that will, if feeding randomly once, end up biting an infectious person: There are ap mosquitoes, and a proportion im of the population carries gametocytes and thus is infectious. This quantity itself is not too informative. However, we consider that the

- proportion b of these mosquitoes that *would* bite an infectious person actually succeed in biting a person

- of these, a proportion s live long enough for the ingested gametocytes to develop into sporozoites and
- of these, a proportion b bite another person.

This gives rise to the funny-looking quantity

$$bsbaimp = b^2 saimp. \tag{5.1}$$

The quantity described by expression (5.1) is actually the number of mosquito bites capable of transmitting malaria as a result of mp people with malaria, or, as Ross states it, the "number of infecting mosquitos which succeed in biting again" (p. 156).

Question 5.b

Translate expression (5.1) to prose, i.e. describe the processes captures by it.

5.2.1 "Laws which Regulate the Amount of Malaria in a Locality"

This modest section title on p. 156 belies the fact that the following eight pages are, for our purpose, the most critical in this volume of almost 800 pages, as he deals with one of the central questions of quantitative epidemiology. In the course of this section, Ross examines the conditions determining whether malaria *increases* or *decreases*. First, though, he introduces two new elements to his model:

1. There are $b^2 saimp$ *potentially infecting events*: Mosquitoes, infected by feeding on mp infected persons, a proportion i of which actually *are* infectious; of these mosquitoes, a proportion s survive to infectiousness, of which a proportion b survive to bite people (each bite on a different person); each of these bites is *potentially infectious*. However, the proportion m of the population already is infected and *re-infection* is, epidemiologically, inconsequential. Therefore, only a proportion $1-m$ of these events—bites on the *susceptible* proportion $1-m$—will result in *new* infections.
2. A proportion r of the infected people clear infection "during the period of observation."

He then states that

> *"[...] the whole number of cases in the locality will have increased or decreased at the end of the period of observation, according to whether $b^2 sai(1-m)mp$, the number of new cases, is greater or less than rmp, the number of recoveries. Thus (neglecting common factors) the change depends upon whether $b^2 sai(1-m)$ is greater or less than r."* (p. 157, second paragraph)

The latter statement seems to imply that

$$\text{The epidemic grows occurs only if } b^2 sai(1-m) > r \tag{5.2}$$

and that

$$\text{The epidemic ebbs only if } b^2 sai(1-m) < r. \tag{5.3}$$

This would follow from the statement before, regarding $b^2sai(1-m)mp$ and rmp, after canceling out the "common factor" mp. If inequalities (5.2) and (5.3) are divided by r, they become

$$\text{Epidemic growth occurs only if } R > 1, \text{ where } R = \frac{b^2sai(1-m)}{r} \tag{5.4}$$

and

$$\text{Epidemic die-out occurs only if } R < 1, \text{ where } R = \frac{b^2sai(1-m)}{r}. \tag{5.5}$$

If we then assume that we are at the very beginning of the outbreak, such that $m \approx 0$, e.g. only *one* infectious case of malaria ($imp = 1$) in a large susceptible population, which also implies that $1-m \approx 1$ and can thus be neglected as factor in the expression, we have

$$R_0^* = \frac{b^2sa}{r}. \tag{5.6}$$

While Eqs. (5.4) and (5.5) characterize the epidemic growth potential given a certain epidemic stage, i.e. a certain level of malaria prevalence in the population, (5.7) characterizes the epidemiological potential of a given situation that is defined by *relative mosquito density* (a), *human biting probability* (b), the *mosquito "infectiousness" proportion* (s), and the *"recovery probability"*. Thus the quantity is—even though not by Ross—labeled R_0^* (0 for the "very beginning").

Interestingly, a different mathematical argument regarding the "epidemic growth potential" becomes apparent if we revisit expression (5.1), i.e. the quantity

$$b^2saimp,$$

which is the number of infectious mosquito bites, and thus infections, resulting from imp infectious people. Setting that original number to again to one, i.e. $imp = 1$, we could write

$$R_0 = b^2sa. \tag{5.7}$$

Expression (5.7) would—like (5.6)—be the number of infections resulting from one "index case". As we will see, this is, at least casually formulated, a definition of the *basic reproduction number.*

Question 5.c

Can you adjudicate the contradiction between the two expressions (5.7) and (5.6) which, purportedly, represent the same quantity?

We will revisit expression (5.7) in the following section when we compare Ross's implicit formulation of that quantity to Macdonald's explicit one.

5.2.2 Final remarks on Ross's modeling contributions

Ross was a copious writer and, obviously, an extremely versatile scientist who is not only credited with discovering the mode of transmission of malaria,[3] but also made important contributions to mathematical modeling of infectious diseases. We have only worked through a few pages of the first edition of his massive volume on "The Prevention of Malaria" [2] which contain relatively primitive mathematical arguments. The second edition of that book contained more sophisticated arguments, which he summarized in a short article [3]. I will briefly comment on some aspects of that paper shortly. A few years later, Ross published a series of papers on *"a priori pathometry"* which, in essence, is a fundamental layout of mathematical (maybe as opposed to statistical = "a posteriori") modeling. Ross's work (as well as Macdonald's, whose work we will encounter in the next section) is more thoroughly examined by Smith et al. [4]. I hope that, reading the latter, you will easily spot inaccuracies such as the statement that

> *"Daniel Bernoulli developed a dynamic model of smallpox transmission and control in 1760."*[4] *[4, p. 2]*

In his "Prevention of Malaria", Ross develops a *difference equation model* of the following form

$$m_{i+1}p = m_i p + b^2 sai(1 - m_i)m_i p - rm_i p, \tag{5.8}$$

for $i \in \{0, 1, 2, \ldots\}$ where the transition from i to $i + 1$ represents a time step, for example, one month; m_0 is the prevalence of malaria at the onset.

Question 5.d

What use could you envision for the recursive equation (5.8)?

Eq. (5.8) represents one of the earliest dynamic transmission models in the literature. We have, in earlier chapters (Chaps. 2 & 3) encountered two models that were more (En'ko's) or less (Hamer's) prior to Ross's model. Ross may not have been aware of these authors; at least, to my knowledge, he mentioned neither in his writings. That would make his contribution even more remarkable and would qualify him as one of the "inventors" of mathematical modeling of infectious diseases.

In his short 1911 paper [3], he takes his model one step further by making the time steps infinitesimally small, i.e. by making his difference equation model into a differential equation model for a "metaxenous disease", i.e. disease requiring two alternate hosts[5] (p. 467):

$$\frac{dz}{dt} = k'z'(p - z) + qz, \tag{5.9}$$

[3] The fairness of Ross being awarded the Nobel Prize for Medicine or Physiology in 1902 for his important discoveries related to malaria transmission has been questioned. Giovanni Battista Grassi, an Italian researcher, has been deemed at least as important for our understanding of malaria as Ross.

[4] We saw in Chap. 1 that Bernoulli's model was an enormous contribution, but *not* a dynamic model.

[5] This is not a modern term.

$$\frac{dz'}{dt} = kz(p'-z')+q'z', \tag{5.10}$$

where z represents the number of infected individuals, for example, people, and z' represents the other involved type of infected host, e.g. mosquitoes. The coefficient q represents changes to the number, such as mortality, etc. Ross defines this as $q = V-1-r-N$, where V incorporates changes in the number of infected due to immigration, emigration, reproduction, and mortality, but which is only defined for the difference equation model. There Ross refers to these quantities as *rates*; however, they are, in that case *proportions*. I believe that his definition of q is incorrect, due to a confusion of rates and proportions, but that does not demean his model. q' is defined equivalently for the other "species". k and k' are *transmission parameters* from one species to the other. Ross then develops the equilibrium density of z, commenting that we "then obtain immediately":

$$z = \frac{kpk'p'-qq'}{kk'p'-kq}. \tag{5.11}$$

Question 5.e

Derive Eq. (5.11) from the system of two differential equations (5.9) and (5.10).

5.3 George Macdonald: Malaria equilibrium beyond Ross

Approximately four decades after Ross, George Macdonald built on Ross's malaria work, among others, to examine the equilibrium of malaria. Macdonald, at the time, was Professor of Tropical Hygiene at the London School of Hygiene and Tropical Medicine and was Director of the Ross Institute of Tropical Hygiene. His paper "The analysis of equilibrium in malaria" [1] is a nice, comprehensive, and very readable epidemiologic overview of malaria. The main text is almost entirely free of mathematical expressions (except for one expression on p. 817), but is based on an interpretation of the mathematical insights gained from the derivation laid out in the Appendix. It contains a typology of malaria (*stable*, *unstable*, *epidemic*) and a "comparison of theory with nature", which is insightful. Here, however, I will devote all my attention to the mentioned Appendix that starts with a notational introduction:

m Density of *Anopheles* mosquitoes relative to humans;
a Number of people a mosquito bites per day;
n Time to completion of the extrinsic cycle (development of sporozoites) after infectious blood meal;
b Proportion of infectious mosquitoes;
h Proportion of the human population receiving infectious mosquito bites per day;
x Proportion of people with parasitemia (malaria parasites in blood);
L Equilibrium proportion of infectious people;

r Proportion of infected people reverting to the unaffected state per day;
t Time in days.

5.3.1 A linear model

Macdonald begins with the demonstration of some previously published results that are based on a linear model, first assuming that h (per-day infection proportion) does not exceed r (per-day recovery proportion):

$$\frac{dx}{dt} = h - rx, \tag{5.12}$$

$$L = \frac{h}{r}, \tag{5.13}$$

$$x = L - (L - x_0)e^{-rt}. \tag{5.14}$$

These are Eqs. (1), (2) and (3), respectively, in the paper. Eq. (5.12) describes the rate of change in the proportion of people who are parasitemic; that change is determined by a *constant* infection rate h and the recovery rate r.

Question 5.f

Why did I refer to (5.12) as a *linear* model?

I will point out issues with this equation shortly (Sect. 5.3.1.1), but let us first accept it to explain Eqs. (5.13) and (5.14).

Eq. (5.13)

L is the equilibrium prevalence of infected people. At equilibrium, the prevalence of infection in people does not change, i.e. $\frac{dx}{dt} = 0$. Therefore, if we set Eq. (5.12) to zero, we can solve for $x^* = L$, the value of x at equilibrium:

$$0 = h - rx^*,$$

$$rx^* = h \text{ (bring } rx^* \text{ over to the other side)}, \tag{5.15}$$

$$x^* = L = \frac{h}{r}. \tag{5.16}$$

Eq. (5.14)

As (5.12) is a linear first order differential equation, it can be solved using well-known methods that are covered in any textbook treating first order linear ordinary differential equations. The equation has to be brought into the form:

$$\frac{dx}{dt} + p(t)x = q(t). \tag{5.17}$$

The solution to (5.17) is

$$x = \frac{\int e^{\int p(t)dt} q(t)dt + c}{e^{\int p(t)dt}}. \tag{5.18}$$

Solution (5.18) may look both miraculous and intimidating, but it is derived relatively easily, though we will not do that here. To use this solution, we let

- $p(t) = r$; while $p(t)$ *could* be a function of time, in our case, it is just a constant.
- $q(t) = h$, also just a constant.

Thus, Eq. (5.12) can be written as

$$\frac{dx}{dt} + rx = h, \tag{5.19}$$

which gives rise to the solution

$$\begin{aligned}
x &= \frac{\int e^{\int r dt} h dt + c}{e^{\int r dt}} \\
&= \frac{h \int e^{rt} dt + c}{e^{rt}} \quad (\int r dt = rt; h \text{ constant}) \\
&= \frac{\frac{h}{r} e^{rt} + c}{e^{rt}} \quad (\int e^{rt} dt = \frac{h}{r} e^{rt}) \\
&= \frac{h}{r} + ce^{-rt} \text{ (dividing numerator by } e^{rt}) \\
x &= L + ce^{-rt} \text{ (using Eq. (5.13)).}
\end{aligned} \tag{5.20}$$

As the last step, to reconstruct Eq. (5.12) we have to find c, which I leave up to you.

Question 5.g

Find c in Eq. (5.20). (*Hint*) Start with $x(0)$.

Using the solution to Question 5.g for c, we can complete the solution for x from Eq. (5.20) as

$$\begin{aligned}
x &= L + ce^{-rt} \\
&= L + (x_0 - L)e^{-rt} \\
&= L - (L - x_0)e^{-rt}.
\end{aligned} \tag{5.21}$$

So we have verified Eq. (5.21).

5.3.1.1 Issues with the model

Before examining the expression for L (Eq. (5.13)), I alluded to some issues with model (5.12). I will now comment on that:

1. The two parameters, h and r, are defined as "proportions per day". Proportions and rates are closely related: Let λ be rate per unit of time, then, as λ gets small, $\lambda \approx 1 - e^{-\lambda}$.
   However, proportions do not correspond well with a differential equation model; the parameters that describe the "flux", say from the infected class to the susceptibles, as r in rx, are rates. Therefore, these parameters should be defined as *rates*.

2. The only term on the right-hand side of Eq. (5.12) that describes the influx into the infected class is h. Macdonald states that h, the "transmission parameter", is constant. As the human risk of malaria infection is a function of the number of infectious *Anopheles* mosquitoes (carrying sporozoites), while that number is a function of the number of infectious people, h, in reality, cannot be constant. However, making simplifying "linearizing" assumptions may be a reasonable step in the solution of a problem. Here, however, not only the rate of the *flux* into the infected class is constant, but also the flux itself. This clearly is *not* a reasonable simplification. As we saw in Chap. 1, Bernoulli recognized the fact that the incidence of an infectious disease is also a function of the number of susceptibles around. In Chap. 3, we examined Hamer's and Soper's focus on that principle. Therefore, the transmission term in model (5.12) should be $(1-x)h$ instead of h; $1-x$ represents the susceptible proportion in the population.

The corrected model (5.12) should therefore be written as

$$\frac{dx}{dt} = h(1-x) - rx. \tag{5.22}$$

The equilibrium value of x, L would therefore also be different.

Question 5.h

Derive the corrected equilibrium value of x according to model (5.22).

With the new equilibrium value of x given by $L = \frac{h}{r+h}$ we see that also Eq. (5) in the paper, stating the equilibrium value of x if "h equals or exceeds r" as

$$L = 1, \tag{5.23}$$

cannot be correct because 1 is only the limiting value of L if h goes to infinity, but r does not. We therefore ignore Eqs. (4) and (6) and go right to the derivation of the expression for the basic reproduction number.

5.3.2 *The "basic reproduction rate of malaria"*

5.3.2.1 *Mosquito survival*

The probability of a mosquito to survive a full day is given by p. Assume that mosquito survival is "memory-less", meaning that the probability to survive from one day to the next, given that it has survived up to that point, is constant. Note that this does not imply that the probability to survive 7 days is the same as surviving 14 days; it only implies that the *conditional survival probability* does not change. This is not a realistic model of mosquito survival, as an age of a mosquito of, say 10 years, would be unlikely, but possible; any entomologist would disqualify such a possibility. But, at the same time, it may be a reasonable model as mosquito mortality may be so dominated by predation and environmental causes over biological aging. A constant conditional survival probability implies a constant mortality rate μ. The probability to "die" on day t, $q(t)$, is then given by the exponential distribution

$$q(t) = \mu e^{-\mu t}. \tag{5.24}$$

Accordingly, the probability to die between day 0 to day 1 is given by the definite integral of (5.24):

$$\begin{aligned}
\int_{t=0}^{1} q(t)dt &= \int_{t=0}^{1} \mu e^{-\mu t} dt, \\
Q &= \mu \int_{t=0}^{1} e^{-\mu t} dt \text{ (μ is a constant)}, \\
&= -\frac{\mu}{\mu} e^{-\mu t}\Big|_0^1 \text{ (integral of $e^{-\lambda t}$ with respect to t)}, \\
Q &= 1 - e^{-\mu} \text{ (probability to die in one day)}, && (5.25) \\
p &= 1 - Q = e^{-\mu} \text{ (probability to survive one day)}. && (5.26)
\end{aligned}$$

The survival probability is simply the complement of the death probability Q, i.e. $1 - Q$. If we consider Eq. (5.26), we can see that we can recover the mortality rate from p as follows:

$$\begin{aligned}
p &= e^{-\mu}, \\
-\mu &= \log(p) \text{ (rearrange, take natural log)}, \\
\mu &= -\log(p) \text{ (multiply by -1)}. && (5.27)
\end{aligned}$$

So, Eq. (5.27) gives us the mortality rate as a function of the daily survival probability. Now, a property of the *exponential distribution* is the fact that the inverse of its parameter μ is its *mean*, i.e. the *mean time of death*. But this is nothing other than the *life expectancy*! Therefore, we get Macdonald's expression (7), i.e. "a mosquito's expectation of life is"

$$\frac{1}{-\log p}. \tag{5.28}$$

5.3.2.2 An important definition

Macdonald then proceeds to present the following definition of the "basic reproduction rate of malaria":

> *"The number of infections distributed in a community as the direct result of the presence in it of a single primary non-immune case."*

He then continues by stating that that *index case* would be infective for $\frac{1}{r}$ days.

Question 5.i

Why would the index case be infectious for $\frac{1}{r}$ days?

Note regarding infected vs infectious

You may have noticed that the use of *being infected* (x) and being *infectious* is somewhat muddled here. While r is defined as the *rate of recovery* from *infection*, a different meaning of r is implied here: rate of recovery from *infectiousness* (carrying sporozoites). This does not diminish the importance of Macdonald's seminal formulation of the basic reproduction number, but it is important to pay attention to such details.

During each of these $\frac{1}{r}$ days, the original case will, "on average", be bitten by m mosquitoes, this is the number of mosquitoes allotted to each person, a time each. Note that a will usually be below 1 (mosquitoes usually do not bite every day). Therefore, there will be

$$\frac{ma}{r} \tag{5.29}$$

opportunities of mosquitoes to become infected by the index case. A proportion p^n of these mosquitoes will survive long enough for *sporozoites* to mature. Mosquitoes that survive to become infectious will survive another $\frac{1}{-\log p}$ days during each of which they will bite a times, infecting a proportion b of the bitten people. Putting this all together, we get

$$\begin{aligned} R_0 &= \frac{ma}{r} \times p^n \times \frac{1}{-\log p} \times a \times b \\ &= \frac{ma^2bp^n}{-r\log p}. \end{aligned} \tag{5.30}$$

The symbol R_0 (= "*R nought*", "*R naught*", or "*R zero*") is now widely accepted as symbol for the *basic reproduction number*, sometimes called the *basic reproductive number* or even *basic reproduction rate* (even though it is clearly *not* a rate).

5.3.3 Comparing Ross's—implicit—and Macdonald's R_0 for malaria

As I pointed out, Ross did not explicitly formulate an expression for R_0 for malaria, but expression (5.7) is clearly implied by his model. It would be interesting to compare, side-by-bide, that expression with Macdonald's explicit expression for R_0, i.e. (5.30).

Table 5.1 Representation of critical quantities in the two expressions for R_0

Quantity	Ross	Macdonald
No. mosquitoes becoming infected (1)	ba	$\frac{am}{r}$
Prop. of (1) becoming infectious (2)	s	p^n
Prop. of (2) succeeding in biting again	b	$\frac{a}{-\log p}$

Let me recall Ross's expression (5.7),

$$R_0 = b^2 sa.$$

Macdonald's expression (5.30), on the other hand, is

$$R_0 = \frac{ma^2bp^n}{-r \log p}.$$

It is natural and legitimate, of course, that every author uses the notation she or he finds most appropriate. Unfortunately, however, Macdonald mostly used the same letters Ross did, but assigned different meanings to them. Some of the quantities represented in Ross's and Macdonald's expression for R_0 are similar, but not exactly equivalent; therefore, the symbols cannot be easily translated. Table 5.1 compares the expression from the respective expressions. A few comments on Table 5.1:

1. Infection of mosquitoes by biting infectious people is captured differently by the two models: Ross incorporates that in b, which is the proportion of mosquitoes biting people–there is just *one* infectious. Macdonald specifies the duration of infectiousness ($\frac{1}{r}$) and applies the biting rate, a, to that time interval (i.e. multiplying the two quantities).
2. The delivery of infectious mosquito bites is also handled differently: Ross captures that by the product of the proportion of infected mosquitoes that become infectious, s, and the proportion biting again, b, giving sb. Macdonald captures the process in more detail as a function of the survival to infectiousness, p^n, the life expectancy, $\frac{1}{-\log p}$, and the biting rate a, $\frac{ap^n}{-\log p}$.
3. What seems to be lacking in both models is the completion of the cycle, i.e. getting all the way to *infectious* people, thus tallying the number of *infectious* people (secondary cases) who result from *one infectious* person (index case). Both expressions only give the numbers of secondary infections due to the index case. However, the assumption that *everybody* who has malaria also has gametocytes in the blood periodically is, for all practical purposes, absolutely reasonable. It means that everybody infected will become infectious. In reality, there will be intervening events, such as death, possibly unrelated to the event, but such events would likely not be very consequential.

Appendix 5.A Answers

5.a To compute the probability that a single released anopheline mosquito will transmit malaria, we have to consider the following events with associated probabilities:

1. The probability that a mosquito will bite a human, which is, by assumption, "4 to 1 against this happening" or $\frac{1}{4} = 0.25$. This quantity is actually not quite useful as such, without making further specifications: As we don't know how old that mosquito is, its probability to bite any human could have a wide range of values (from close to 0 to 0.25 in this case). We therefore have to define that probability as the *probability to bite a human during its remaining life time*. We call this parameter b (see following text).
2. The probability that the mosquito, *if* biting a human, will bite just the one we are most interested in, i.e. the one with *gametocytes* in her blood. This conditional probability, assuming that all humans are equally attractive to mosquitoes (which, undoubtedly, many will dispute), is $\frac{1}{p} = 0.001$, where p is the size of the local population (see text).

Putting these two probabilities together, using the basic properties of probabilities, we get

$$\begin{aligned}\Pr(A \cap B) &= \Pr(A) \times \Pr(B|A)\\ &= b \times \frac{1}{p}\\ &= 0.25 \times 0.001\\ &= 0.00025.\end{aligned}$$

The number 0.00025 is, of course, the same answer Ross himself gives to that question ($\frac{1}{4000}$). *Comments:*

- $\Pr(A \cap B)$ is the joint probability of events A and B, i.e. the probability that *both* event A *and* B happen.
- A is the event that a mosquito will bite a human and
- B is the event that mosquito bites specific individual if it bites a human.

5.b The quantity $b^2 saimp$ can be translated as follows:

1. There are p people.
2. Of these, a proportion of m have malaria.
3. Of these, a proportion i carry gametocytes, thus there is a proportion im of people who are capable of transmitting malaria to mosquitoes.
4. There are a mosquitoes per person, thus ap mosquitoes.
5. Of these, proportion b will succeed taking a blood meal.
6. Therefore, there will be $apimb$ blood meals of mosquitoes that will infect mosquitoes, i.e. newly infected mosquitoes.
7. Of these infected mosquitoes, a proportion i will survive to allow sporozoites to develop and thus to become infectious.

8. Finally, of those new infectious mosquitoes, again, a proportion b will succeed to take another blood meal, to infect a susceptible person.

5.c The problem with the first expression for the *epidemic growth parameter*,

$$R_0^* = \frac{b^2 sa}{r},$$

stems from its derivation from a kind of, but not quite, difference equation model which is implied by Ross describing the scenario (quote on page 92) where he states that the number of cases "[...] will have increased or decreased at the *end of the period of observation*." So, while the original case is subject to recovery, all the secondary cases, which are infected by the *full* original infectious case are not subject to recovery; in fact, in this context, recovery is irrelevant for quantifying the epidemiological potential. Now, to be sure, Ross did not come up with this expression of R_0^*; I constructed it from a suggestive mathematical argument laid out in the quote on page 92 and inequalities (5.2) and (5.3). Also, I will disprove my statement that recovery is irrelevant for R_0 in the next section, but the context there is different. As to the expression for R_0 (5.7),

$$R_0 = b^2 sa,$$

we tally the number of *infected humans* that result from the first infectious (for mosquitoes!) case of malaria ($imp = 1$) as

- a human is bitten by ab mosquitoes which become infected,
- of which s survive to the development of sporozoites,
- of which a proportion b succeed in susceptible humans,
- presumably, all those *infected* become *infectious* to mosquitoes.

The second expression (5.7) is more appropriate: The quantification of the epidemic potential has to enumerate the secondary cases at the same stage of the epidemic process we started to keep track. Here this means we have to count the number of *infectious* humans that result from the *infectious index case*.

5.d Ross's recursive model of malaria transmission can be used to *simulate* a malaria epidemic and to see what happens over time. This could be easily implemented on a personal computer, but back in Ross's time this involved more work. The difference equation model also offers a way to easily calculate equilibrium values. This can be done by forcing the model not to change any more, by setting $m_{i+1} = m_i = m$ and solving the equation for m. This helps to investigate the *endemic* level of malaria which will result from certain parameter values, i.e. values for b, s, a, i, and r.

5.e Equilibrium of the system (5.9) and (5.10) implies that both equations are zero, i.e. "nothing changes". First, we can solve Eq. (5.9) for z':

$$\begin{aligned} 0 &= k'z'(p-z) + qz, \\ k'z'(p-z) &= -qz \text{ (bring } kz(p'-z') \text{ to the other side, multiply by } -1), \\ z' &= \frac{qz}{k'(p-z)} \text{ (divide by } k'(p-z)). \end{aligned} \tag{5.31}$$

Next, similarly solve (5.10) for $z = \frac{q'z'}{k(p'-z')}$ and substitute (5.31) for z':

$$\begin{aligned}
z &= \frac{q'z'}{k(p'-z')} \\
&= \frac{q'\frac{qz}{k'(p-z)}}{k(p' - \frac{qz}{k'(p-z)})} \\
&= \frac{q'\frac{qz}{k'(p-z)}}{k(\frac{p'k'(p-z)-qz}{k'(p-z)})} \text{ (manipulate the expression in the denominator)} \\
&= \frac{q'qz}{k(p'k'(p-z)-qz)} \text{ (cancel } k'(p-z)\text{)}, \\
zkp'k'(p-z) - kqz^2 &= q'qz \text{ (multiply by } k(p'k'(p-z)-qz)\text{)}, \\
kp'k'(p-z) - kzq &= q'q \text{ (divide by } z\text{)}, \\
z &= \frac{kk'pp' - qq'}{kp'k' - kq} \text{ (rearrange)}.
\end{aligned}$$

We have thus verified expression (5.11).

5.f Differential equation (5.12) ("model") is *linear* because all the terms are *linear*, i.e. it does not contain products of variables–in this case that would be mosquitoes and people. In fact, the rate of infection of people is, by assumption, constant and thus independent of infection prevalence in mosquitoes. This has important implications for solving this equation.

5.g To find c we simply have to look at the "beginning of time", i.e. where $t = 0$. Using that in $x = L + ce^{-rt}$, we get

$$\begin{aligned}
x_0 &= L + ce^{-r0}, \\
x_0 &= L + c \text{ (because } e^0 = 1\text{)}, \\
c &= x_0 - L \text{ (rearrange)}.
\end{aligned}$$

5.h If we set Eq. (5.22) to zero, calling L the equilibrium value of x, we get:

$$\begin{aligned}
0 &= h(1-L) - rL, \\
h(1-L) &= rL, \\
h - hL &= rL, \\
h &= rL + hL \text{ (adding } hL \text{ to both sides)}, \\
h &= L(r+h) \text{ (factoring } L\text{)}, \\
\frac{h}{r+h} &= L.
\end{aligned}$$

Therefore,

$$L = \frac{h}{r+h}. \tag{5.32}$$

5.i The answer to this question is, again, related to the *exponential distribution*. Here we are dealing not with mortality, but with reversion to the unaffected state, which is driven by the parameter r. In analogy to the argument leading to the expression for the life expectancy (= average time to death), we are looking for the *average time infectious* = *average time to reversion*. Based on the distribution for the time to reversion

$$u(t) = re^{-rt}, \tag{5.33}$$

we easily find the average time to reversion (i.e. the average time infectious) by simply inverting the parameter r, i.e. $\frac{1}{r}$.

Let me comment on the use of the *exponential distribution*. I have gotten in some "muddy water" here because I used the exponential distribution in the statistical sense, and we have noted before that there is no room for probability in the *realm of deterministic models*. However, there is this natural connection between linear differential equations, that can describe, for example, a failure time process (such as mortality, etc.) and the exponential distribution (see, for example, Eq. (5.20), etc.). You may have noticed, though, that Macdonald, like many other authors, casually mix statistical concepts with the probability-incompatible deterministic world of differential equation models.

References

[1] G. Macdonald, The analysis of equilibrium in malaria, Tropical Diseases Bulletin 49 (9) (1952) 813–829.
[2] R. Ross, The Prevention of Malaria, Dutton, 1910.
[3] R. Ross, Some quantitative studies in epidemiology, Nature 87 (1911) 466–467.
[4] D.L. Smith, K.E. Battle, S.I. Hay, C.M. Barker, T.W. Scott, F.E. McKenzie, Ross, Macdonald, and a theory for the dynamics and control of mosquito-transmitted pathogens, PLoS Pathog 8 (4) (2012) e1002588.

M. Bartlett (1949), N.T. Bailey (1950, 1953) and P. Whittle (1955): Pioneers of stochastic transmission models

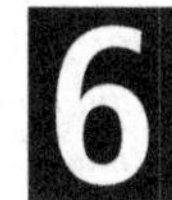

Contents

6.1 Introduction: Stochastic transmission models

The papers discussed so far [4–8], even though often evoking the idea of events happening, such as "subjects" becoming infected or being removed from the infectious class, are intrinsically deterministic treatments of transmission processes. In his introductory paragraph to his paper "A simple stochastic epidemic" [1], Bailey states that:

> *"The mathematical theory of epidemics has usually been confined to the consideration of 'deterministic' models as, for example, in the work of Kermack & McKendrick (1927 and later) and Soper (1929). That is, it has been assumed that,*

A Historical Introduction to Mathematical Modeling of Infectious Diseases. DOI: 10.1016/B978-0-12-802260-3.00006-7

for given numbers of susceptible and infectious individuals and given infection and removal rates, a certain definite number of fresh cases would arise in a given time. In fact, as is well known, a considerable degree of chance enters into the conditions under which fresh infections take place, and it is clear that for a more precise analysis we ought to take these statistical fluctuations into account. In short, we require 'stochastic' models to supplement existing deterministic ones."

Question 6.a

Why do you think deterministic models became so much more popular than stochastic models (this is, by the way, still the case)?

We have, of course, already encountered the works of Kermack and McKendrick [7] and Soper [8] in previous chapters. It is still clear that the predominant body of literature on transmission models is devoted to deterministic models, but stochastic considerations are in some instances very important. The stochastic treatment of infectious disease transmission requires an entirely different set of mathematical tools and also heavily relies, naturally, as chance is involved, on statistical concepts.

Besides the paper by Kermack & McKendrick (Chap. 4), the papers discussed in this chapter may be, for the non-mathematician (as myself), the most difficult ones to fully appreciate. I will crisscross papers from three authors, Maurice Stevenson Bartlett (1910–2002), Norman T.J. (Thomas John) Bailey (1923–2007), and finally, Peter Whittle (1927–). The four papers I will discuss are closely related and, at least partially, cross-reference each other. Even though Bartlett's contribution was published first and is the most general one in scope, I will begin with Bailey's 1950 paper entitled "A simple stochastic epidemic" [1], mostly to accustom the reader to the topic. I will then move on to Bartlett's 1949 "Some evolutionary stochastic processes" [3], but will narrowly focus on the two sections at the very end of the paper that deal with transmission processes. This will prepare us for Bailey's second paper which was published three years after the first one (1953) and is entitled "The total size of a general stochastic epidemic" [2]. We will then finish this chapter by examining the comment on the latter paper by Whittle from the year 1955 [9].

6.2 Bailey: A simple stochastic transmission model

This paper [1] may be suited as an introduction to the topic because the model treated here is the simplest. Bailey assumes an infectious agent that leads to chronic infection, but has no other detrimental effect.

6.2.1 Deterministic approach

The model could be written like Eq. (4.34) of the "Kermack & McKendrick model" (Chap. 4, p. 71):

$$\frac{dx}{dt} = -\kappa xy.$$

To be consistent with Bailey, the following notation is used:

$$\frac{dy}{dt} = -\beta yx, \tag{6.1}$$

where y now, confusingly, is used for the number susceptible (at time t) and x for the number infectious. n represents the original size of the susceptible population into which one infectious individual is introduced. β is used for the transmission parameter or the "infection rate". If the time scale is defined as $t^* = \beta t$ and the "*" is omitted, the model can be written as

$$\frac{dy}{dt} = -y(n - y + 1). \tag{6.2}$$

As the transmission parameter has been integrated into the time measure, it vanishes from the equation. Note that the number of infectious must be the number of originally susceptible, n, minus the number of currently susceptible, y, plus one, because otherwise the index case would be omitted. Thus, $x = n - y + 1$. Also, for $t = 0$ (start of transmission process) $y = n$. After rearranging, this equation appears as an example of a so-called *Bernoulli differential equation*:

$$\frac{dy}{dt} + (n + 1)y = y^2. \tag{6.3}$$

This was not "our" Bernoulli (Daniel, Chap. 1), but his uncle Jacob on his father's side. The general form of a Bernoulli differential equation is

$$\frac{dy}{dt} + p(t)y = q(t)y^n, \tag{6.4}$$

where $p(t)$ and $q(t)$ are continuous functions of t, and n is a real number. The method for solving a Bernoulli differential equation can be described as follows:

1. Let $v = y^{1-n}$ and $\frac{dv}{dt} = (1 - n)y^{-n}\frac{dy}{dt}$.
2. Solve this expression for $\frac{dy}{dt}$ by dividing both sides by $(1 - n)$ and by y^{-n} which is equivalent to multiplying by y^n. This yields $\frac{dy}{dt} = \frac{dv}{dt}\frac{1}{1-n}y^n$.
3. Divide Eq. (6.4) by y^n, which results in

$$\begin{aligned} y^{-n}\frac{dy}{dt} + y^{-n}\,p(t)\;y\;y^{-n} &= q(t), \\ y^{-n}\frac{dv}{dt}\frac{1}{1-n}y^n + y^{1-n}p(t) &= q(t)\;(y\;y^{-n} = y^{1-n}), \\ \frac{dv}{dt} + v\;p(t) &= q(t) \end{aligned} \tag{6.5}$$

$(y^{-n} \times y^n = 1$; substitute v for $y^{1-n})$.

4. Eq. (6.5) is a *linear differential equation* which can be solved for v. The solution can then be expressed in terms of y, using $y = v^{1/(1-n)}$.

Let us now turn from the general case to our problem at hand, i.e. Eq. (6.3), which represents Eq. (6.4) with $n = 2$, $p(t) = n+1$, and $q(t) = 1$. Invoking the steps outlined above, we first define $v = y^{-1} = \frac{1}{y}$ and $\frac{dv}{dt} = -\frac{1}{y^2}\frac{dy}{dt}$ and, accordingly, solve for $\frac{dy}{dt} = -\frac{dv}{dt}y^2$. This expression for $\frac{dy}{dt}$ is used in Eq. (6.3):

$$\begin{aligned}
\frac{dy}{dt} + (n+1)y &= y^2, \\
-\frac{dv}{dt}y^2 + (n+1)y &= y^2, \\
-\frac{dv}{dt} + (n+1)\frac{1}{y} &= 1, \\
-\frac{dv}{dt} + (n+1)v &= 1, \\
\frac{dv}{dt} - (n+1)v &= -1.
\end{aligned} \tag{6.6}$$

The linear differential equation (6.6) has the following solution (this can be read in any text dealing with differential equations):

$$\begin{aligned}
v &= \frac{-\int e^{-\int (n+1)dt}dt}{e^{-\int (n+1)dt}} \\
&= \frac{-\int e^{-(n+1)t}dt}{e^{-(n+1)t}} \text{ (the expression } (n+1) \text{ is constant)} \\
&= \frac{-\frac{1}{N+1}e^{-(n+1)t} + C}{e^{-(n+1)t}} \text{ (the fraction results} \\
&\text{from the integration of the exponential function)} \\
&= \frac{1}{n+1} + Ce^{(n+1)t} \text{ (dividing both terms of the numerator by } e^{-(n+1)t} \text{ or,} \\
&\text{equivalently, multiplying them by } e^{(n+1)t}\text{)} \\
&= \frac{1 + (n+1)Ce^{(n+1)t}}{n+1}.
\end{aligned} \tag{6.7}$$

Eq. (6.7) is a solution for v, but we need a solution for y. We do know, however, that $y = \frac{1}{v}$; y therefore is simply the right-hand side of (6.7) inverted, i.e.

$$\begin{aligned}
y &= \frac{1}{v} \\
&= \frac{1}{\left(\frac{1+(n+1)Ce^{(n+1)t}}{n+1}\right)} \\
&= \frac{n+1}{1 + (n+1)Ce^{(n+1)t}}.
\end{aligned} \tag{6.8}$$

As we know the initial condition for y, $y(0) = y_0 = n$, this Bernoulli equation is a *initial value problem*, and we can solve for C. As $y(0) = n$, we can write:

$$n = \frac{n+1}{1 + (n+1)C} \text{ (time } t = 0\text{, so the exp falls away),}$$

$$\begin{aligned}
1+(n+1)C &= \frac{n+1}{n} \text{ (multiply by right denominator and divide by } n\text{)},\\
(n+1)C &= \frac{n+1}{n} - 1 \text{ (subtract 1 from both sides)},\\
(n+1)C &= \frac{1}{n} \text{ (note that } \frac{n+1}{n} - 1 = \frac{n+1}{n} - \frac{n}{n} = \frac{n+1-n}{n}\text{)},\\
C &= \frac{1}{n(n+1)} \text{ (divide both sides by } (n+1)\text{)}. \qquad (6.9)
\end{aligned}$$

We can plug this solution for C into Eq. (6.8) to obtain

$$\begin{aligned}
y &= \frac{n+1}{1+(n+1)Ce^{(n+1)t}}\\
&= \frac{n+1}{1+(n+1)\frac{1}{n(n+1)}e^{(n+1)t}} \text{ (plug-in solution for } C\text{)}\\
&= \frac{n+1}{1+\frac{1}{n}e^{(n+1)t}} \text{ (rearrange)}\\
&= \frac{n(n+1)}{n+e^{(n+1)t}} \text{ (multiply numerator and denominator by } n\text{)}. \qquad (6.10)
\end{aligned}$$

Question 6.b

What exactly was achieved by Eq. (6.10)?

6.2.2 Stochastic approach

The fundamental assumptions are the same as for the deterministic model, but now we wish to reflect on a situation where at time t there is not always a particular "number" of susceptible, infectious and, usually, removed subjects.

Question 6.c

Why did I set the word *number* in quotes?

Therefore, the number of each type (i.e. susceptible, infectious, etc.) of individuals at time t is not a suitable outcome for a stochastic model. Instead, we will model the probability that there are a certain number of, say susceptible, individuals at time t. The notation Bailey uses is $p_r(t)$, the probability that there are r susceptible individuals at time t. Note that in this simple model the probability that there are s infectious individuals at time t is simply $o_s(t) = 1 - p_r(t)$. We therefore do not bother with that—complimentary—probability ($o_s(t)$).

Instead of a differential equation of the numbers of susceptibles (Eq. (6.2)), we formulate a differential equation for the probabilities $p_r(t)$. As Bailey states [1, p. 196]:

> *"Then the usual treatments shows that the epidemic process is characterized by the stochastic differential-difference equations:"*

$$\frac{dp_r(t)}{dt} = (r+1)(n-r)p_{r+1}(t) - r(n-r+1)p_r(t) \quad (r = 0, 1, 2, \ldots, (n-1)), \tag{6.11}$$

$$\frac{dp_n(t)}{dt} = -np_n(t). \tag{6.12}$$

This is one of numerous, similarly unhelpful, statements that are scattered throughout the literature, the kind of which ultimately motivated this book. Some explanations are therefore in order. What Eqs. (6.11) and (6.12) capture is the change over time in the probability that, at time t, r susceptibles remain. That probability, $p_r(t)$, can change by two means:

1. If there are r susceptibles and one becomes infected, there will be fewer susceptibles (exactly *one* less) and $p_r(t)$ will decline. The rate of decline will therefore be at the rate at which this (i.e. one becoming infected) happens. That rate is $r(n-r+1)$ (see Question 6.d). This rate must be weighted by the probability that there actually are r susceptibles, which is, of course, $p_r(t)$. One important detail regarding these rates is the fact that they are expressed as "per t", but that t is not time in, e.g., *days*, but in *time* $\times\beta$ (see remarks in Sect. 6.2.1).
2. If there are $r+1$ susceptibles and one becomes infected, there will be r susceptibles, thereby increasing $p_r(t)$. This increase happens at a rate $(r+1)(n-r)$ which, again, has to be weighted by $p_{r+1}(t)$.

Question 6.d

Why is the rate at which new infections arise when there are r susceptibles $r(n-r+1)$ and $(r+1)(n-r)$ if there are $r+1$ susceptibles?

Eqs. (6.11) and (6.12) are not directly solvable, but can be solved with the help of Laplace transforms which are powerful tools in mathematics and engineering. There are many introductions to the topic available.[1] Bailey gives the following expression for the Laplace transform and its inverse:

$$\mathcal{L}(\phi(t)) = \phi^*(\lambda) = \int_0^\infty e^{-\lambda t}\phi(t)dt, \tag{6.13}$$

$$\phi(t) = \frac{1}{2\phi i}\int_{c-i\infty}^{c+i\infty} e^{\lambda t}\phi^*(\lambda)d\lambda, \tag{6.14}$$

[1] Many of these I had to resort to myself!

where $\int_{c-i\infty}^{c+i\infty} \equiv \lim_{w\to\infty} \int_{c-iw}^{c+iw}$; note that λ is a complex number. A common symbol used for the Laplace transform is $\mathcal{L}(\cdot)$; Bailey uses an asterisk for the transformation and q_r for the Laplace transform of $p_r(t)$. For someone not familiar with Laplace transforms, Eqs. (6.13) and (6.14) may be quite intimidating, but in many cases, the transform and its inverse do not have to be calculated, but can be looked-up in tables. The transforms of Eqs. (6.11) and (6.12), however, have to be calculated.

Question 6.e

Calculate the Laplace transform of (6.11). To that end, both sides of the equation have to be multiplied by $e^{-\lambda t}$ and integrated with respect to t from 0 to ∞ (improper integral). Pay attention to the boundary conditions (expression (7) in [1]):

$$p_r(t) = \begin{cases} 1 & \text{for} \quad r = n, \\ 0 & \text{for} \quad r < n. \end{cases}$$

The Laplace transform of the right-hand side of Eq. (6.11) is obtained simply by switching out the ps for qs, where the latter are the Laplace transforms of the former, i.e. $q_r = \int_0^\infty e^{-\lambda t} p_r(t)dt$:

$$\begin{aligned} &\int_0^\infty e^{-\lambda t}(r+1)(n-r)p_{r+1}(t) - r(n-r+1)p_r(t)dt \\ &\quad = (r+1)(n-r)q_{r+1} - r(n-r+1)q_r. \end{aligned} \tag{6.15}$$

Writing out the Laplace transform of the whole Eq. (6.11) (both sides), we can combine the answer to Question 6.e and Eq. (6.15) to get

$$\begin{aligned} \lambda q_r &= (r+1)(n-r)q_{r+1} - r(n-r+1)q_r, \\ q_r\,(\lambda + r(n-r+1)) &= (r+1)(n-r)q_{r+1} \text{ (adding } r(n-r+1)q_r \text{ to both sides} \\ &\quad \text{and factoring } q_r), \\ q_r &= \frac{(r+1)(n-r)}{\lambda + r(n-r+1)} q_{r+1} \\ &\quad \text{(dividing both sides by } \lambda + r(n-r+1)). \end{aligned} \tag{6.16}$$

Similar procedures can be used to obtain the Laplace transform of Eq. (6.12). First, for the left-hand side we have:

$$\begin{aligned} \int_0^\infty e^{-\lambda t}\frac{dp_n(t)}{dt}dt &= e^{-\lambda t}p_n(t)\big|_0^\infty + \lambda\int_0^\infty e^{-\lambda t}p_n(t) \\ &= \lim_{t\to\infty} e^{-\lambda t}p_n(t) - e^{-\lambda 0}p_n(0) + \lambda q_n \\ &= \lambda q_n - 1. \end{aligned} \tag{6.17}$$

A few remarks regarding Eq. (6.17):

- $\lim_{t\to\infty} e^{-\lambda t} p_n(t) = 0$ because $\lim_{t\to\infty} e^{-\lambda t} = 0$;
- $e^{-\lambda 0} = 1$ and $p_n(0) = 1$—see "boundary conditions" and therefore $-e^{-\lambda 0} p_n(0) = -1$;
- $\lambda q_0 = \lambda \int_0^\infty e^{-\lambda t} p_n(t)$ because the integral is nothing but the Laplace transform of $p_n(t)$; the λ in front is due to the fact that the derivative of $\int_0^\infty e^{-\lambda t}$ with respect to t is $\lambda \int_0^\infty e^{-\lambda t}$, and that is used for the integration-by-parts (see the answer to Question 6.e).

The Laplace transform of the right-hand side of Eq. (6.12) is, by definition

$$-\int_0^\infty e^{-\lambda t} n p_n(t) dt = -n q_n. \tag{6.18}$$

Equating the right-hand sides of (6.17) and (6.18) we obtain the following equation (Eq. (6.12), Laplace-transformed):

$$\begin{aligned} -n q_n &= \lambda q_n - 1, \\ q_n (\lambda + n) &= 1 \text{ (subtracting } \lambda q_n \text{ and multiplying by } -1), \\ q_n &= \frac{1}{\lambda + n} \text{ (dividing by } \lambda + n). \end{aligned} \tag{6.19}$$

So we have Laplace-transformed Eqs. (6.11) and (6.12), presented here together (Eqs. (6.16) and (6.19)):

$$\begin{aligned} q_r &= \frac{(r+1)(n-r)}{\lambda + r(n-r+1)} \times q_{r+1}, \\ q_n &= \frac{1}{\lambda + n}. \end{aligned}$$

Question 6.f

If you consider these two Laplace-transformed Eqs. (6.11) and (6.12), i.e. Eqs. (6.16) and (6.19), does a way to calculate q_r become obvious?

In the full expression for q_r, Eq. (6.133), that is developed in the answer to Question 6.f, the numerator can be rearranged, such that we get a product of the form $n \times (n-1) \times \ldots \times r \times (r+1)$ and one of the form $(n-r) \times (n-r-1) \times \cdots \times 1$. The latter could be rewritten as a factorial, i.e.

$$(n-r)! = (n-r) \times (n-r-1) \times \cdots \times 1.$$

The former product does not go "all the way", i.e. from n to 1; in that case, it could have been written as $n!$. Unfortunately, it runs only from n to $(r+1)$. However, if $n!$ is divided by $r \times (r-1) \times \cdots \times 1 = r!$, we rid ourselves of that part of the factorial we do not need. Accordingly, the numerator of the right-hand side of Eq. (6.133) can be written as

$$(n-r)!\frac{n!}{r!} = \frac{(n-r)!n!}{r!}. \tag{6.20}$$

Table 6.1 Duplicity of some factors in the denominator of the right-hand side of Eq. (6.22)

	$n=8$	$n=9$
j	$j \times (8-j+1)$	$j \times (9-j+1)$
1	$1\times(8-1+1)=8$	$1\times(9-1+1)=9$
2	$2\times(8-2+1)=14$	$2\times(9-2+1)=16$
3	$3\times(8-3+1)=18$	$3\times(9-3+1)=21$
4	$4\times(8-4+1)=20$	$4\times(9-4+1)=24$
5	$5\times(8-5+1)=20$	$5\times(9-5+1)=25$
6	$6\times(8-6+1)=18$	$6\times(9-6+1)=24$
7	–	$7\times(9-7+1)=21$

The denominator of the right-hand side of Eq. (6.133) can be written as

$$\prod_{j=1}^{n-r+1} \lambda + (n-j+1)\, j. \tag{6.21}$$

Combining (6.20) and (6.21), we obtain Bailey's Eq. (9) (bottom of p. 196):

$$q_r = \frac{\frac{(n-r)!\, n!}{r!}}{\prod_{j=1}^{n-r+1} \lambda + j\,(n-j+1)}, \quad \text{for } 0 \le r \le n. \tag{6.22}$$

Bailey notes that

> "*... if $r \ge \frac{1}{2}\,(n+1)$, then the factors in the denominator are all different, while if $r < \frac{1}{2}\,(n+1)$ some of them are repeated." (top of p. 197)*

This is easier to understand with an example. For that purpose, let first $n = 8$ and pick two values for r, such as $r = 6$ and then $r = 3$.

According to Bailey, no factors should be repeated for $r = 6$, since then $6 > \frac{1}{2}$ $(n+1) = 4.5$ (see quote from top of p. 197, [1]). In fact, if $r = 6$, the factors run, for $j = 1$ to $j = n - r + 1 = 8 - 6 + 1 = 3$, shown in the first three lines of the column for "$n = 8$" of Table 6.1; all three factors are unique. If $r = 3$, however, Bailey predicts some factors of the denominator (6.21) to be duplicate, because $3 < \frac{1}{2}\,(n+1) = 4.5$. If $r = 3$, the factors run, for $j = 1$ to $j = n - r + 1 = 8 - 3 + 1 = 6$, shown in the first six lines of the first column of Table 6.1: Factors 3 and 6 are identical (= 18), as are factors 4 and 5 (= 20); all three factors are unique. This is because the first factor of the product $j \times (n - j + 1)$ increases with j, while the second factor decreases; the same product will be obtained, for example, with $3 \times (8 - 3 + 1) = 18$ and with $6 \times (8 - 6 + 1) = 18$. If n is odd, for example, $n = 9$, the largest factor, here 25, is not duplicated. If two factors are duplicated, they can be expressed as a square (e.g. 24^2).

After these, somewhat tedious derivations, we need to remind ourselves of what we are—or, rather, what Bailey is—trying to achieve: We are trying to find a way to calculate $p_r(t)$, the probability that there are r susceptibles left at time t. What we just accomplished is to find a way to calculate the Laplace transform of $p_r(t)$, q_r.

It should therefore be easy to obtain an expression for $p_r(t)$ by simply finding the inverse Laplace transform of q_r; most important Laplace transforms and their respective inverses are well-known and tabulated. Unfortunately, there is no (at least not an easy) way to define the inverse Laplace transform of Eq. (6.22). Bailey identifies the solution to this problem by suggesting to use a partial fraction decomposition; that procedure transforms the fraction

$$q_r = \frac{\frac{(n-r)!\,n!}{r!}}{\prod_{j=1}^{n-r+1} \lambda + j\,(n-j+1)}$$

into something like this:

$$\frac{(n-r)!\,n!}{r!}\left(\frac{A_1}{\lambda+n} + \frac{A_2}{\lambda+2\,(n-1)} + \cdots + \frac{A_{n-r+1}}{(n-r+1)\,r}\right). \tag{6.23}$$

The challenge here is to find the numerators $A_1, A_2, \ldots, A_{n-r+1}$. I will briefly illustrate how to achieve this with a simple example, letting $n = 3$ and $r = 3$. Accordingly,

$$\begin{aligned} q_r = q_3 &= \frac{\frac{(4-3)!\,4!}{r!}}{(\lambda+1\,(4-1+1))\,(\lambda+2\,(n-2+1))} \\ &= \frac{4}{(\lambda+4)\,(\lambda+6)}. \end{aligned} \tag{6.24}$$

Note that the product in the denominator runs from 1 to $4-3+1 = 2$. So the goal here is to express the fraction $\frac{4}{(\lambda+4)\,(\lambda+6)}$ as partial fraction of the form:

$$4 \times \left[\frac{A_1}{(\lambda+4)} + \frac{A_2}{(\lambda+6)}\right]. \tag{6.25}$$

The 4 in front of the partial fraction (6.25) is from the numerator in (6.24). The numerators A_1 and A_2 can be determined in three steps:

1. Consider equation $\frac{1}{(\lambda+4)\,(\lambda+6)} = \frac{A_1}{(\lambda+4)} + \frac{A_2}{(\lambda+6)}$ from (6.24) and (6.25), after dividing by 4. Multiply both sides by $(\lambda+4)\,(\lambda+6)$, which gives $1 = A_1\,(\lambda+6) + A_2\,(\lambda+4)$.
2. Set $\lambda = -4$: $1 = A_1\,(-4+6) + A_2\,(-4+4)$ which allows us to solve for $A_1 = \frac{1}{2}$.
3. Set $\lambda = -6$: $1 = A_1\,(-6+6) + A_2\,(-6+4)$ which allows us to solve for $A_2 = -\frac{1}{2}$.

This leads to the expression

$$\begin{aligned} q_3 &= \frac{4}{2\,(\lambda+4)} - \frac{4}{2\,(\lambda+6)} \\ &= \frac{2}{(\lambda+4)} - \frac{2}{(\lambda+6)} \\ &\quad \text{(dividing numerators and denominators by 2).} \end{aligned} \tag{6.26}$$

The inverse Laplace transform of these simple fractions can now be easily found. As the numerators of the two fractions in Eq. (6.26) are constants, they can be ignored for the inverse Laplace transform and we have to transform only $\frac{1}{(\lambda+4)}$ and $-\frac{1}{(\lambda+4)}$. Looking up in a table for Laplace transforms, we find for the inverse Laplace transform

$$\frac{1}{2}\mathcal{L}^{-1}\left(\frac{1}{(\lambda+4)}\right)=\frac{1}{2}\,e^{-4t}. \tag{6.27}$$

Similarly, the negative Laplace transform of the second fraction is $\frac{1}{2}e^{-6t}$. Putting together, we have found a closed-form expression for $p_3(t)$:

$$p_3(t)=\frac{1}{2}\,e^{-4t}+\frac{1}{2}\,e^{-6t}. \tag{6.28}$$

Plugging-in a value for t, we now can calculate $p_3(t)$ and see that after, say, 5 "days" (remember that the transmission parameter is integrated into the time measure), the probability of 3 susceptibles remaining is virtually zero.

Even though this is by no means the end of Bailey's paper [1], I will leave it at that. By now we have developed a basic understanding of some important concepts and strategies that can be used when dealing with stochastic transmission models. Before revisiting Bailey, specifically his paper [2] that followed the current paper after a few years, I will briefly discuss part of an article by Bartlett [3]. This should help us to better understand Bailey's follow-up paper.

6.3 M.S. Bartlett: Infectious disease transmission as stochastic process

Bartlett's paper entitled "Some evolutionary stochastic processes" [3] was a highly innovative contribution to the statistical theory of stochastic processes. An infectious transmission is not the main focus of the paper; Bartlett deals with a wide range of topics, ranging from insurance risk to demographic processes. We jump right into the relevant passages, i.e. Sect. 7 which is entitled "Mixed processes in epidemiology" (p. 225).

6.3.1 Fundamentals

The fact that we skip the earlier parts of this paper may be justified by the fact that they are not directly relevant to the issues this book is dealing with, but we have to pay the price for jumping right into the figurative "cold water". The second sentence of the section, for example, states:

> *"The probabilities of transitions for multiplicative processes are proportional to the number of individuals existing, this giving rise to the operator $\frac{\partial}{\partial z}$." (p. 225, lower half)*

This, to the unprepared, must seem exceedingly obscure. To understand, we have to introduce the *probability-generating function* which can be very useful in this context. This is actually also the topic that Baley is taking up in his paper [1] right after the position in the text where we abandoned it; it is, however, not presented there in a very helpful manner.

A probability-generating function is a series of the form

$$G(z) = \sum_{x=0}^{\infty} p(x)z^x = E(z^x) \tag{6.29}$$

where $p(x)$ is the probability density function of x and $E(\cdot)$ is the expectation or the expected value.

> The expected value $E(X)$ is an important concept in statistics. It is defined as:
>
> $$E(X) = \int_x xf(x)dx \text{ (integral over the whole domain of } x). \tag{6.30}$$
>
> In the case of a discrete random variable, the above integral becomes a sum, and the probability distribution function $f(x)$ becomes a probability. The expected value is nothing but the mean.

This definition of the probability-generating function implies that they are only relevant to discrete random variables that only take non-negative integers as their values.

One of the useful properties of the probability-generating function is the following:

$$p(x) = \frac{G(z)^{(x)}(0)}{x!}, \tag{6.31}$$

i.e. the xth derivative of $G(z)$, evaluated at 0, retrieves the probability $p(x)$. As we are interested in the probability of certain quantities, in particular the number of infectious and susceptible individuals, over time and we may have ideas of how these probabilities change with time, the derivatives of the probability density function with respect to time may be of interest. We will now use Bartlett's notation: Let X denote the random variable representing the number of infectious individuals and Y the random variable representing the number still susceptible. It is presently more common to switch these labels of infectious (Y) and susceptible individuals (X), but the use of Bartlett's original notation will make it easier to follow the paper. For full consistency, these random variables should be explicitly indexed by time, i.e. $X(t)$ and $Y(t)$, but I omit the time index to remain as close as possible to Bartlett. Specific values for X and Y are written as x and y. To approach the probability mass distribution of X and Y, it is essential that we characterize how these random variables can change at time t.

> **Question 6.g**
>
> Characterize how X and Y can change at time t if infected individuals become immediately infectious (as in the "Kermack & McKendrick" model) and eventually become "removed" from infectiousness by recovery (or death).

As shown in the answer to Question 6.g, there are only two types of processes in a "Kermack & McKendrick-type" model; Bartlett considers one additional process,

Table 6.2 **Possible random transitions**

Type of transition	Average rate	Operator
$zw \to w^2$	λ	$\frac{\partial^2}{\partial z \partial w}$
$w \to 1$	μ	$\frac{\partial}{\partial w}$
$1 \to z$	ν	1

corresponding to "influx of susceptibles" by either immigration or reproduction. This corresponds to $y \to y + 1$. The three described processes happen at the following rates:

1. New infections are driven by the transmission parameter λ and, assuming a "mass action" principle, arise at a rate $xy\lambda$. The concept of mass action plays an important role in infectious disease modeling, even though originating from chemistry. We first encountered this in Soper's work (Chap. 3).
2. Infectious individuals recover at a rate μ, such that, given x infectious individuals, the rate of infectious subjects being removed is $x\mu$.
3. New susceptibles are recruited at a rate ν.

Here, we are dealing with a probability-generating function of two random variables:

$$\Pi(z, w) = \sum_{x,y} p(x, y)\, z^y w^x. \tag{6.32}$$

$p(x, y)$ is the joint probability density function of x and y; this would be the same as $p(x)p(y)$ if x and y were independent. As transmission processes are, however, inherently dependent, these two random variables are *not* independent. Now we are ready for Table 6.2 (top of p. 226 [3]).

The meaning of the left-most column of Table 6.2 is relatively easy to grasp on an *intuitive* level: z represents susceptible, w infectious. In terms of the probability-generating function, if one individual becomes infectious, there is one less susceptible. This can be represented by

$$z^y w^x \to z^{y-1} w^{x+1}$$

which is, somewhat symbolically or, as Bartlett puts it, as an "idealized scheme", expressed as $zw \to w^2$ (first row). If one infectious individual recovers, one infectious individual "vanishes" as he/she is not longer taking part in the process. This can be represented as $w \to 1$ (second row). Finally, if a new susceptible is recruited, $1 \to z$ (last row).

The second column represents the rate parameters driving the respective transition. The last column, labeled "operator", is a little more difficult to understand. But before continuing to explore this, we jump right into Bartlett's Eq. (49) which is the partial derivative of the probability-generating function with respect to time.

6.3.2 The change in the probability-generating function over time

The partial derivative of the probability-generating function (6.32) with respect to time captures how it changes over time:

$$\frac{\partial \Pi}{\partial t} = \lambda(w^2 - zw)\frac{\partial^2 \Pi}{\partial z \partial w} + \mu(1-w)\frac{\partial \Pi}{\partial w} + v(z-1)\Pi \tag{6.33}$$

where Π is used for $\Pi(z, w)$. This equation, in fact, contains all the elements from Table 6.2. To really understand the rationale, we may need some explanations. To approach this issue, let us revisit the probability-generating function (6.32),

$$\Pi(z, w) = \sum_{x,y} p(x, y)\, z^y w^x .$$

Even though the time dependence of the probability-generating function is not explicitly stated, it is quite obvious that the transmission process that is captured here *is* time-dependent.

Question 6.h

How does (6.32) change over time (i.e. what actually changes)?

As we have seen in the answer to Question 6.h, the probabilities $p(x, y)$ associated with $z^y x^w$ change over time. The processes that invoke these changes in $p(x, y)$ are listed in Table 6.2: Transmission, removal/recovery and recruiting of new susceptibles. I will now comment on how this relates to Eq. (6.33).

First, however, I would like to highlight an important, even crucial, aspect of my approach. The stochastic model we are dealing with here represents a *Markov Chain*. A Markov chain is a random process that is characterized by states that can be enumerated—here this would be combinations of x and y—and the state transitions of which do *not* depend on the past, but only on the *current* state of the system. In our case, we are dealing with a *continuous-time Markov chain* because events do not happen in discrete time steps. There is a large body of literature and theory on Markov chains. As a non-mathematician I have only shallow knowledge of this like, possibly, some of my readers. My goal is to demonstrate that, nevertheless, using basic mathematical principles, we can attain a deep understanding of this and other important texts.

Change in the probability-generating function due to new infections: The first term

To characterize the change in the probability-generating function which is due to *new infections* at time t, it is helpful to first focus on one specific scenario, i.e. if there are exactly x infectious and y susceptible individuals. Note that events never happen simultaneously, so there will always be just *one* new infection etc.

1. The probability that, at time t there are *exactly* x infectious and y susceptible individuals is, by definition

$$p(x, y), \tag{6.34}$$

which, as mentioned before, should be indexed by time, but the time index has been omitted for convenience. This probability can also be interpreted as the weight assigned to the contribution to the *total change* in the probability-generating function that is due to this particular case (x infectious and y susceptible individuals).

2. The rate at which, given x infectious and y susceptible individuals, a new individual is infected is determined by the rate of transmission, driven by the rate parameter λ (first row, middle column of Table 6.2). Assuming "mass action" (see Eq. (6.1)), that rate of transmission is

$$yx\lambda. \tag{6.35}$$

3. If, given this situation, a new individual is infected, it results in *one less* susceptible $(y - 1)$ and *one more* infectious individual $(x + 1)$. The term $z^y w^x$ of the probability-generating function is changed to $z^{y-1}w^{x+1}$. The *amount* of change in the probability-generating function due to new infection thus is

$$z^{y-1}w^{x+1} \ (\textit{new} \text{ state}) - z^y w^x \ (\textit{old} \text{ state}). \tag{6.36}$$

4. The total amount of change in the probability-generating function at time t due to new infection if there are x infectious and y susceptible individuals is therefore given by the product of (6.34), (6.35) and (6.36),

$$p(x, y) \times yx\lambda \times \left(z^{y-1}w^{x+1} - z^y w^x\right). \tag{6.37}$$

To tally up the total amount of change in the probability-generating function due to new infection, we simply have to sum (6.37) over all possible x, y-combinations:

$$\sum_{x,y} p(x, y)\, yx\lambda \left(z^{y-1}w^{x+1} - z^y w^x\right). \tag{6.38}$$

Expression (6.38) can be rearranged in the following way:

$$\begin{aligned}
&= \sum_{x,y} p(x, y)\, yx\lambda \left(w^2 z^{y-1}w^{x-1} - zwz^{y-1}w^{x-1}\right) \\
&\quad \text{(using } z^{y-1}w^{x+1} = w^2 z^{y-1}w^{x-1} \text{ and } z^y w^x = zwz^{y-1}w^{x-1}\text{)} \\
&= \sum_{x,y} p(x, y)\, yx\lambda \left(w^2 - zw\right) z^{y-1}w^{x-1} \\
&\quad \text{(factoring } z^{y-1}w^{x-1}\text{)} \\
&= \lambda \left(w^2 - zw\right) \sum_{x,y} p(x, y)\, yx\, z^{y-1}w^{x-1} \qquad (6.39) \\
&\quad \text{(} w \text{ and } z \text{ are constants; } (w^2 - zw) \text{ can thus be} \\
&\quad \text{multiplied with the sum)}
\end{aligned}$$

$$= \lambda(w^2 - zw)\frac{\partial^2\Pi}{\partial z \partial w} \tag{6.40}$$

(see explanation below).

Some brief explanations on how we got from Eq. (6.39) to Eq. (6.40):

1. The partial derivative of the probability-generating function with respect to z is:

$$\begin{aligned} \frac{\partial\Pi}{\partial z} &= \frac{\partial \sum_{x,y} p(x,y)\, z^y w^x}{\partial z} \\ &= \sum_{x,y} p(x,y)\, yz^{y-1} w^x. \end{aligned} \tag{6.41}$$

2. Taking the partial derivative of expression (6.41) with respect to w is:

$$\begin{aligned} \frac{\partial^2\Pi}{\partial z \partial w} &= \frac{\partial \sum_{x,y} p(x,y)\, yz^{y-1} w^x}{\partial z} \\ &= \sum_{x,y} p(x,y)\, xyz^{y-1} w^{x-1}. \end{aligned} \tag{6.42}$$

We have thus justified the substitution of $\frac{\partial\Pi^2}{\partial z \partial w}$ for $\sum_{x,y} p(x,y)\, xyz^{y-1} w^{x-1}$ to get from Eq. (6.39) to Eq. (6.40).

These derivations prove that Eq. (6.40) and thus the first term of the right-hand side of Eq. (6.33), the partial derivative of the probability-generating function with respect to time, represents the change in the probability-generating function over time that is due to new infections. Bartlett refers to this as a "mixed" process because it is driven by the product of two variables, x and y.

Change in the probability-generating function due to removal of infectious subjects: The second term

To characterize the change in the probability-generating function due to the *removal* of infectious individuals, we can proceed as we did in the previous section and, first, characterize the rate at which infectious individuals are removed and then quantify the resulting change in the probability-generating function:

1. The rate at which infectious individuals are removed is driven by the rate parameter μ (second row, middle column of Table 6.2) and by the number infectious (x). That rate of removal is thus given by

$$x\mu. \tag{6.43}$$

2. The removal of one infectious individual results in *one less* infectious individual ($x - 1$), but leaves the number of susceptibles unchanged (y). Accordingly, the term $z^y w^x$ of the probability-generating function is changed to $z^y w^{x-1}$. The *amount* of change in the probability-generating function due to new infection thus is

$$z^y w^{x-1} - z^y w^x. \tag{6.44}$$

3. The total change in the probability-generating function due to removal of infectious individuals if there are x infectious and y susceptible individuals is therefore given by the product of (6.34), (6.43) and (6.44),

$$p(x, y) \times x\mu \times \left(z^y w^{x-1} - z^y w^x\right). \tag{6.45}$$

Using similar reasoning as in the previous section, we can sum Eq. (6.45) over all values of x and y,

$$\sum_{x,y} p(x, y)x\mu \left(z^y w^{x-1} - z^y w^x\right) \tag{6.46}$$

and rearrange as follows:

$$\begin{aligned}\sum_{x,y} p(x, y)x\mu \left(z^y w^{x-1} - z^y w^x\right) &= \sum_{x,y} p(x, y)x\mu \left(z^y w^{x-1} - wz^y w^{x-1}\right)\\ &= \sum_{x,y} p(x, y)x\mu \,(1-w)\, z^y w^{x-1}\\ &= \mu\,(1-w) \sum_{x,y} p(x, y)xz^y w^{x-1}\\ &= \mu\,(1-w)\frac{\partial \Pi}{\partial w} \qquad (6.47)\\ &\quad \text{(noting that } \sum_{x,y} p(x, y)xz^y w^{x-1} = \frac{\partial \Pi}{\partial w}\text{)}\end{aligned}$$

This proves that the second term of the partial derivative of the probability-generating function with respect to time, i.e. the left-hand side of Eq. (6.33), which is identical to Eq. (6.47), represents the change in the probability-generating function over time that is due to removal of infectious subjects.

Bartlett refers to this kind of process as "multiplicative" because it is proportional to one variable, here x.

Change in the probability-generating function due to immigration: The third term

Finally, change in the probability-generating function can also be caused by *recruitment* of new susceptibles (immigration, reproduction). Again, we can proceed as we did in the previous two sections dealing with the first and second terms of the right-hand side of Eq. (6.33), but I leave this to you:

Question 6.i

Derive the third term of the right-hand side of Eq. (6.33).

As shown in the answer to Question 6.i, the third term of the partial derivative of the probability-generating function with respect to time, i.e. the left-hand side of

Eq. (6.33) represents the change in the probability-generating function over time that is due to recruitment of susceptible individuals. Bartlett refers to this kind of process as "additive" because it is not proportional to any variable.

Bartlett observes that similar equations can be developed for other models. If, instead of an $S \to I \to R$ model, according to which infection results in immediate infectiousness, infectiousness is preceded by a latent phase (infected, but not yet infectious) an $S \to E \to I \to R$ ("SEIR") model results, where "E" represents the latent phase. For such a model, the first term on the right-hand side of Eq. (6.33) will be replaced by

$$\lambda(ww_1 - zw)\frac{\partial^2 \Pi}{\partial z \partial w} + \lambda_1(w - w1)\frac{\partial \Pi}{\partial w_1} \tag{6.48}$$

where w_1 corresponds to the latent state and λ_1 represents the parameter driving the transition from the latent to the infectious state ($E \to I$).

However, as Bartlett points out,

> *"[u]nfortunately the exact solution of these equations is less simple." (middle of p. 226)*

By "less simple" he is, in fact, insinuating "not possible" which seems unfortunate indeed because of the amount of time we have spent trying to understand Eq. (6.33). In modern research in infectious disease modeling, however, the solution of (partial) differential equations is often not the primary goal. Rather,

> *"[if] this is not feasible theoretically, the more pedestrian method of investigating the solution by random numbers may have to be used." (top of p. 227)*

Given our easy access to powerful computation, numerical solutions are often the main tool of exploring transmission models.

Question 6.j

How would you implement Bartlett's transmission model?

6.3.3 Mean value equations

We will now turn to the last aspect of Bartlett's paper: A characterization of the change in the *expected* number of susceptibles and infectious individuals at time t. Bartlett uses lower case notation (x,y) to denote the expected number. He arrives at these expressions as follows:

> *"[...] we may differentiate [Eq. (6.33)] in turn with respect to w and z. Putting $z = w = 1$, we then obtain the two exact equations*
>
> $$\frac{\partial x}{\partial t} = \lambda E(XY) - \mu x,$$
> $$\frac{\partial y}{\partial t} = -\lambda E(XY) - \nu."$$
>
> *(lower half of p. 226)*

Using $E(\cdot)$ for the expected value instead of lower case notation, these equations become:

$$\frac{\partial E(X)}{\partial t} = \lambda E(XY) - \mu E(X), \quad (6.49)$$

$$\frac{\partial E(Y)}{\partial t} = -\lambda E(XY) - \nu. \quad (6.50)$$

I will provide a few explanations of how Bartlett arrived at these expressions as well as some comments, focusing on Eq. (6.49). How does differentiation of $\frac{\partial \Pi}{\partial t}$ with respect to w become $\frac{\partial E(X)}{\partial t}$? Differentiation of the left-hand side of Eq. (6.33) with respect to w results in

$$\begin{aligned}\frac{\partial \frac{\partial \Pi}{\partial t}}{\partial w} &= \frac{\partial^2 \Pi}{\partial t \partial w} \\ &= \frac{\partial \frac{\partial \Pi}{\partial w}}{\partial t} \quad (6.51)\\ &\text{(change in order of partial derivatives, } \textit{Schwartz' theorem}\text{).}\end{aligned}$$

This simply allows us to first determine the partial derivative with respect to w and set $w = z = 1$; we are then left with a partial derivative with respect to time; if, in fact, this were $\frac{\partial E(X)}{\partial t}$, we would have verified the left-hand side of (6.51). Accordingly, we just have to check whether $\frac{\partial \Pi}{\partial w}$ is actually $E(X)$:

$$\begin{aligned}\frac{\partial \Pi}{\partial w} &= \sum_{x,y} p(x,y)\, x\, z^y w^{x-1} \text{ (see Eq. (6.47))} \\ \left.\frac{\partial \Pi}{\partial w}\right|_{z=w=1} &= \sum_{x,y} p(x,y)\, x \text{ (setting } z = w = 1) \\ &= \sum_x x \sum_y p(x,y) \text{ (rearranging)} \\ &= \sum_x p(x) x \text{ (note that } \sum_y p(x,y) = p(x)) \quad (6.52)\\ &= E(X) \text{ (right-hand side of (6.52) is the definition of } E(X)).\end{aligned}$$

The partial derivative of the right-hand side of (6.33) with respect to w needs to be approached in a slightly different manner. The right-hand side of (6.33) is

$$\lambda(w^2 - zw)\frac{\partial^2 \Pi}{\partial z \partial w} + \mu(1 - w)\frac{\partial \Pi}{\partial w} + v(z - 1)\Pi.$$

These three terms are of the form fg where both f and g are functions of w and z, respectively. If, for example, we want to get the partial derivative of fg with respect to x, we have to use the product rule ($\frac{\partial fg}{\partial w} = \frac{\partial f}{\partial w} g + \frac{\partial g}{\partial w} f$). Applying this to the first term, the following results:

$$\frac{\partial \lambda (w^2 - zw) \frac{\partial^2 \Pi}{\partial z \partial w}}{\partial w} = \lambda (2w - 1) \frac{\partial^2 \Pi}{\partial z \partial w} + \lambda (w^2 - zw) \frac{\partial^3 \Pi}{\partial z \partial w^2} \tag{6.53}$$

$$= \lambda (2 - 1) \sum_{x,y} p(x, y)\, xyz^{y-1} w^{x-1} \tag{6.54}$$

$$+ \lambda (1 - 1) \sum_{x,y} p(x, y)\, x(x - 1) yz^{y-1} w^{x-2}$$

$$\left. \frac{\partial \lambda (w^2 - zw) \frac{\partial^2 \Pi}{\partial z \partial w}}{\partial w} \right|_{w=z=1} = \lambda (2 - 1) \sum_{x,y} p(x, y)\, xy \tag{6.55}$$

$$= \lambda\, E(XY). \tag{6.56}$$

A few comments regarding Eqs. (6.53) to (6.56):

1. In Eq. (6.53), we take the partial derivative with respect to w of the first term of the left-hand side of Eq. (6.33), using the product rule (right-hand side).
2. In Eq. (6.54) that partial derivative is evaluated using the full expression of the probability-generating function.
3. In Eq. (6.55), Eq. (6.54) is evaluated at $w = z = 1$: $(2w - 1)$ thus becomes $(2 \times 1 - 1) = 1$ and $(w^2 - wz) = (1 - 1) = 0$; because of the latter result, the whole second term falls away (multiplied by 0).
4. The sum on the right-hand side of Eq. (6.55) is nothing but $E(XY)$ or $\mathrm{Cov}(X, Y)$, the covariance of X and Y.

Question 6.k

Treat the second and third expression of the sum on the right-hand side of Eq. (6.33) as we just treated the first expression.

In the answer to Question 6.k we have completed the verification of Eq. (6.49). Eq. (6.50) is obtained similarly.

Even though these mean value equations provide a link to deterministic models, their use is not quite evident. However, if many outbreaks suiting the model could be observed, these equations may offer a way to parameter estimation. But this will not be discussed here.

Bartlett then enters a brief discussion of three articles by Hamer, Soper and Kermack & McKendrick [6–8]—we have extensively analyzed these papers (Chaps. 3 and 4). A more general, relatively non-technical discussion of the stochastic measles model follows. But we are, more or less, well prepared to revisit Bailey's work, this time examining a follow-up paper to the one already examined [1].

6.4 Bailey revisited: Final size of a stochastic epidemic

This paper [2] is based on a model which is somewhat different from the "simple stochastic model" discussed in Sect. 6.2 which dealt with Bailey's earlier paper [1]. The starting point is, in fact, very familiar to us: the "Kermack & McKendrick" model (p. 178, Eq. (1)). The only difference is the—by now familiar—scaling of time by the transmission parameter, like in [1], so that the transmission parameter does not show up in the model equations.

6.4.1 *Reference to Bartlett*

In this paper, Bailey commences his stochastic treatment of "Kermack & McKendrick" with the probability-generating function or, rather, the partial differential equation of the probability-generating function—this is where I left of the earlier Bailey's paper [1] to get an introduction by Bartlett. Bailey directly refers to Barlett's formulation. Remember that Bartlett's model was different from the classical "Kermack & McKendrick" model in that it allowed for reproduction, i.e. replenishment of the susceptibles. Bailey introduces the model's stochastic version as follows:

> *"Then on the assumption of homogeneous mixing of the susceptibles and infectious individuals in circulation the probability of one new infection taking place in time dt is $xydt$, while the probability of one infected person being removed from circulation in time dt is $\rho y dt$. Let $p_{rs}(t)$ be the probability that at time t there are r susceptibles still uninfected and s infectious individuals in circulation. Let us assume that the epidemic is started by the introduction of a infectious cases into a population of n susceptibles." (bottom of p. 178)*

The partial differential equation for the probability-generating function corresponding to this model is (Eqs. (2) and (3), top of p. 179):

$$\frac{\partial \Pi}{\partial t} = (v^2 - uv)\frac{\partial^2 \Pi}{\partial u \partial v} + \rho(1-v)\frac{\partial \Pi}{\partial v}, \tag{6.57}$$

$$\begin{aligned} \Pi &= \sum_{r=0}^{n}\sum_{s=0}^{n+a} u^r v^s p_{rs} \\ &= \sum_{r,s} u^r v^s p_{rs}. \end{aligned} \tag{6.58}$$

This should look very familiar as this is, except for small differences in notation, equivalent to Eq. (6.33) in Sect. 6.3.

Question 6.I

How does Eq. (6.57), other than in notation, differ from the partial differential equation for the probability-generating function (6.33)?

The Laplace transform of the partial differential equation (6.57) is given by

$$(v^2 - uv)\frac{\partial^2 \Pi^*}{\partial u \partial v} + \rho(1-v)\frac{\partial \Pi^*}{\partial v} - \lambda \Pi^* + u^n v^a = 0 \tag{6.59}$$

where

$$\Pi^* = \sum_{r,s} u^r v^s q_{rs}. \tag{6.60}$$

Like before in Sect. 6.2, q is the Laplace transform of $p(t)$ and the "*" accent also indicates a Laplace transform. In particular,

$$q_{rs} = \int_0^\infty e^{-\lambda t} p_{rs}(t) dt. \tag{6.61}$$

The following boundary condition holds:

$$p_{na}(0) = 1. \tag{6.62}$$

This condition says that, at time $t = 0$, i.e. the very beginning of the epidemic, we know with certainty (probability 1) that there are n susceptibles and a infectious individuals. In order to follow Bailey's argument, we have to assume that

$$\left(\frac{\partial \Pi}{\partial t}\right)^* = \sum_{r,s} u^r v^s \int_0^\infty e^{-\lambda t} dp_{rs}. \tag{6.63}$$

Note that $\left(\frac{\partial \Pi}{\partial t}\right)^* \neq \frac{\partial \Pi^*}{\partial t} = 0$. The latter part is true because Π^* is not a function of time t (time has been "integrated out" by the Laplace transformation), and therefore, a partial derivative with respect to t is zero.

On the other hand, $\left(\frac{\partial^2 \Pi}{\partial u \partial v}\right)^* = \frac{\partial^2 \Pi^*}{\partial u \partial v}$ and $\left(\frac{\partial \Pi}{\partial v}\right)^* = \frac{\partial \Pi^*}{\partial v}$. This can be verified by writing out Π and Π^* as sums.

We can then apply what we did in the answer to Question 6.e to obtain

$$\begin{aligned}
\left(\frac{\partial \Pi}{\partial t}\right)^* &= \sum_{r,s} u^r v^s \int_{t=0}^\infty e^{-\lambda} dp_{rs} \\
&= \sum_{r,s} u^r v^s \lambda q_{rs} \text{ (again, using integration by parts—see below)} \\
&= \lambda \Pi^* - u^r v^s.
\end{aligned} \tag{6.64}$$

The expression $-u^r v^s$ can be explained as follows: Remember that $\left(\frac{\partial \Pi}{\partial t}\right)^*$—as long as we are willing to accept the assumption stated in (6.63)—is the sum $\sum_{r,s} u^r v^s \int_0^\infty e^{-\lambda t} dp_{rs}$. Let me examine two types of terms in that sum (summands) more closely:

1. For $r \neq n, s \neq a$: Using, again, integration by parts we get

$$\begin{aligned} u^r v^s \int_0^\infty e^{-\lambda t} dp_{rs}(t) &= u^r v^s e^{\lambda t} p_{rs}(t)\big|_0^\infty + \lambda \int_0^\infty e^{-\lambda t} p_{rs}(t) u^r v^s dt \\ &= 0 + \lambda q_{rs}. \end{aligned}$$

Note that $u^r v^s$ can be treated like a constant because it is independent of time t. Also, $u^r v^s e^{-\lambda t} p_{rs}(t)\big|_0^\infty = 0$ because, when letting $t = \infty$, the expression vanishes ($e^{-\infty} = 0$), and for $t = 0$ it vanishes because $p_{rs}(0) = 0$ unless $r = n, s = a$.

2. For $r = n, s = a$:

$$\begin{aligned} u^n v^a \int_0^\infty e^{-\lambda t} dp_r(t) &= u^n v^a e^{-\lambda t} p_{na}(t)\big|_0^\infty + \lambda \int_0^\infty e^{-\lambda t} p_{na}(t) u^r v^s dt \\ &= -u^n v^a + \lambda q_{na}. \end{aligned}$$

Here, $\lim_{t\to\infty} u^n v^a e^{-\lambda t} p_{na}(t) = 0$, because $\lim_{t\to\infty} e^{-\lambda\infty} = 0$ but $\lim_{t\to 0} u^n v^a e^{-\lambda t} \times p_{na}(t) = u^n v^a$, because $p_{na}(0) = 1$ and the term has to be subtracted. Carried over to the right side of the equation, the $-$sign turns into a $+$sign.

Bailey continues that, by *equating coefficients* of $u^r v^s$, the following recurrence equations are obtained:

$$\begin{aligned} (r+1)(s-1)q_{r+1,s-1} - \{s(r+\rho)+\lambda\} q_{rs} + \rho(s+1)q_{r,s+1} &= 0, \quad (6.65) \\ -\{a(n+\rho)+\lambda\} q_{na} + 1 &= 0 \quad (6.66) \end{aligned}$$

for $0 < r + s \leq n + a, 0 \leq n, 0 \leq s \leq n + a$. By definition, all q_{rs} for which r and/or s are outside of this range are 0.

Equating coefficients, in this context, indicates the following technique:

Equating coefficients

Consider the following expression:

$$\sum_{r,s} A_{rs} u^r v^s = \sum_{r,s} B_{rs} u^r v^s \quad (6.67)$$

and assume that u and v can assume any real value. Then Eq. (6.67) implies that, for all r, s, $A_{rs} = B_{rs}$.

Let me construct a simple example:

$$A_{21}u^2v^1 + A_{22}u^2v^2 + A_{12}u^1v^2 = B_{21}u^2v^1 + B_{22}u^2v^2 + B_{12}u^1v^2. \quad (6.68)$$

Choose values for the As, etc., for example, $A_{21} = 1$, $A_{22} = 3$, and $A_{12} = 2$; also, set $u = 2$ and $v = 1$. The left-hand side of (6.68) then becomes

$$1 \times 4 \times 1 + 3 \times 4 \times 1 + 2 \times 2 \times 1 = 20.$$

Obviously, if we choose the Bs to be the same as the As with the same subscripts then the right-hand side must also be 20; we could, however, also say $A_{12} = 10$ and both A_{21} and A_{22} are zero, and the right-hand side would still be the same (20). However, if different values for u and v are chosen, the left-hand side and the right-hand side will not be the same. So only if the As and corresponding Bs, associated with any $u^r v^s$ are the same, Eq. (6.68) will always hold—if in doubt, you can try it out.

Eq. (6.67) can be rewritten as

$$\sum_{r,s} A_{rs} u^r v^s - \sum_{r,s} B_{rs} u^r v^s = 0 \tag{6.69}$$

which would similarly indicate that $A_{rs} = B_{rs}$, or $A_{rs} - B_{rs} = 0$. Accordingly, if, instead, we have

$$\sum_{r,s} A_{rs} u^r v^s - \sum_{r,s} B_{rs} u^r v^s - \sum_{r,s} C_{rs} u^r v^s = 0, \tag{6.70}$$

we can say that, for all r, s, $A_{rs} = B_{rs} + C_{rs}$, or $A_{rs} - B_{rs} - C_{rs} = 0$.

Question 6.m

Use Eq. (6.59) to derive the recurrence relationship (6.65) and (6.66).

Having these recursive solutions for the q_{rs}, we could apply the inverse Laplace transform and, from that, calculate the corresponding $p_{rs}(t)$. This may, however, be quite cumbersome, mostly because of the necessary partial fraction decomposition (see page 116). Bailey remarks on this issue that

> *"[t]here seems to be considerable difficulty in handling such expressions in a compact and convenient way to give, for example, epidemic completion times or the stochastic epidemic curve showing the rate of change with respect to time of the average total number of removals at any instant." [2, p. 179]*

However, he points out that focusing on the total size of the epidemic, the problem would be much simplified.

Question 6.n

What values of r and s would be relevant for figuring out the probability distribution function of the *final epidemic size*?

If we focus on the "final size", i.e. the probability of a given size, the quantity of interest becomes $P_w = \lim_{t\to\infty} p_{n-w,0}(t)$ and the following mathematical argument can be developed:

$$\begin{aligned} P_w &= \lim_{t\to\infty} p_{n-w,0}(t) && (6.71)\\ &= \lim_{\lambda\to 0} \lambda q_{n-w,0} && (6.72)\\ &= \lim_{\lambda\to 0} \rho q_{n-w,1} && (6.73)\\ &= \rho f_{n-w,1} && (6.74) \end{aligned}$$

where $f_{n-w,1} = \lim_{\lambda\to 0} q_{n-w,1}$.

Bailey presents Eq. (6.72) without any explanation, but it is justified by the *final value theorem* that is actually precisely stated by (6.72), i.e.

$$P_w = p_{n-w,0}(\infty) = \lim_{\lambda\to 0} \lambda q_{n-w,0}. \quad (6.75)$$

What this really means is that the probability of w individuals being infected during the course of the epidemic—which certainly will be over when time approaches infinity—equals the limit of the Laplace transform of $p_{n-w,0}(t)$, $q_{n-w,0}$, multiplied by λ when λ goes to 0. Conveniently, if we set $r = n - w$, $s = 0$, and $\lambda = 0$ in Eq. (6.65), we obtain

$$q_{rs} = \rho q_{r,1}. \quad (6.76)$$

This relationship is used in Eqs. (6.73) and (6.74). Note that the recurrence equations (6.65) and (6.66) also apply to f_{rs}:

$$\begin{aligned} (r+1)(s-1) f_{r+1,s-1} - \{s(r+\rho)\} f_{rs} + \rho(s+1) q_{r,s+1} &= 0, && (6.77)\\ -\{a(n+\rho)\} q_{na} + 1 &= 0, && (6.78) \end{aligned}$$

or, by rearranging Eqs. (6.77) and (6.78),

$$\begin{aligned} f_{na} &= \frac{1}{a(n+\rho)}, && (6.79)\\ f_{rs} &= \left((r+1)(s-1) f_{r+1,s-1} + \rho(s+1) q_{r,s+1}\right) / \left(s(r+\rho)\right). && (6.80) \end{aligned}$$

This achieves a direct path from $f_{n,1}$, which can be obtained using the recurrence equations (6.79) and (6.80), to P_w, avoiding the partial fraction decomposition that would be necessary otherwise. Bailey then continues with a somewhat obscure "simplification" of f_{rs} which may be valid, but is of unclear use. He then introduces an alternative approach that I will briefly describe in Sect. 6.4.2. Instead, we will work an example that is reflected in Table 1 (p. 182).

Question 6.o

Would you now have the means to calculate the final size probabilities? If so, how would you do it? Assume that, like in Bailey's calculations, there is only one index case, i.e. $a = 1$.

Using the algorithm described in the answer to Question 6.o, the final size probabilities can be calculated, more or less easily. Bailey certainly had no computer at his disposal (maybe a mechanical calculator). Automatic computation clearly simplifies these calculations enormously.

Bailey presents results of calculations for three different magnitudes of n: 10, 20 and 40, both in graphical (Figs. 1–3, p. 181) and in tabular form, as average outbreak sizes (p. 182). These calculations can be reconstructed using the algorithm described in the answer to Question 6.o (online supplement). In conclusion of this paragraph he writes:

> *"There is no obvious analogue of the Threshold Theorem derived by Kermack & McKendrick (1927) for the deterministic case." (p. 182, first paragraph)*

We will revisit this statement in the next section (on Whittle).

6.4.2 Household outbreaks and parameter estimation

I will finish the analysis of Bailey's paper by, somewhat superficially, discussing his analysis of *household outbreaks*. These outbreaks are in no fundamental way different from the outbreaks we just considered; they are simply small and, therefore, numerically more easily to handle. Let us now return to the alternative method alluded to the previous Sect. 6.4.1. Bailey writes that

> *"I am indebted to Dr F.G. Foster for suggesting to me the alternative approach of considering the succession of population states represented by the points (r, s). Thus the progress of the epidemic can be regarded as a random walk from the point (n, a) to the points $(n - w, 0)$ $w = 0, 1, \ldots, n$, with an absorbing barrier at $r = 0$, and where the possible transitions from (r, s) are*

$$(r, s) \rightarrow (r - 1, s + 1), \text{ occurring with probability } r/(r + \rho), \quad (6.81)$$

$$\text{and } (r, s) \rightarrow (r, s - 1), \text{ occurring with probability } \rho/(r + \rho)." \quad (6.82)$$

> *(p. 180, lower half—the expressions are not numbered in Bailey's paper)*

This suggest that these *conditional* probabilities can be directly calculated.

Question 6.p

Why am I referring to conditional probabilities? What do $r/(r + \rho)$ and $\rho/(r + \rho)$ represent?

This consideration of the epidemic process implies a *Markov process* because each transition *only* depends on the current state, i.e. the current values of r and s and not on their histories. Bailey continues that

> *"Foster's general formula for P_w can now be written down almost immediately simply by considering the sum of the probabilities of all possible paths from (n, a) to $(n - w, 0)$."*

I admire Bailey for his impressive ability to write down the following expression "almost immediately", but lack the patience with his unwillingness to offer a helping hand to those among us who sport less ingenious mathematical minds. He offers the following expression:

$$P_w = \frac{\rho^{a+w}}{\rho+n-w} \frac{\binom{n}{w}}{\binom{n+\rho}{w}} \sum_{\alpha} (\rho+n)^{-\alpha_0} (\rho+n-1)^{-\alpha_1} \cdots (\rho+n-w)^{-\alpha_w}, \quad (6.83)$$

"where the summation is over all compositions of $a+w-1$ into $w+1$ parts such that $0 \leq \alpha_i < a+i-1$ for $0 \leq i \leq w-1$ and $1 \leq \alpha_w \leq a+w-1$." At least to me, that seemed utterly obscure at first. Here is an attempt to explain this expression which, in fact, is erroneous (see below).

Foster's formula

Consider the example from the answer to Question 6.o: the size of the susceptible "population" is $n = 10$ and the outbreak is started by one infectious individual, i.e. $a = 1$.

Further assume that $w = 2$, i.e. we are interested in the probability that the outbreak size is 2, i.e. two infections beside the index case. Using Foster's transition probabilities (6.81) and (6.82), to get from one "point", e.g. (5, 1) to another one, e.g. (2, 0) along a specific path, e.g. *via* (3, 3), the corresponding transition probabilities have to be multiplied. By "point" (5, 1) I am referring to the state in which there are 5 susceptibles and 1 infectious individual. As shown in Fig. 6.1 (red edges in online figure) there is more than one path from (5, 1) to (3, 0) which represents the desired outcome with 2 having become infected during the course of the outcome ($5 - 2 = 3$).

To illustrate, let me first focus on one of these paths: from (5, 1) diagonally down to the right to (3, 4) (until two have become infected without anyone being removed) and from there horizontally to the left (all infectious recovering without anyone else becoming infected—marked by fat edges, red in online figure). The corresponding transition probabilities, using (6.81) and (6.82), are shown in the figure:

$$P_{2,1} = \frac{5}{5+\rho} \frac{4}{4+\rho} \frac{\rho}{3+\rho} \frac{\rho}{3+\rho} \frac{\rho}{3+\rho} \quad (6.84)$$

$$= \frac{5 \times 4}{(5+\rho)(4+\rho)} \frac{\rho^3}{(3+\rho)^3} \quad (6.85)$$

$$= \frac{\rho^{2+1} 5!}{(5-2)!} \frac{1}{5+\rho} \frac{1}{4+\rho} \frac{1}{(3+\rho)^3} \quad (6.86)$$

$$= \frac{\rho^{w+a} n!}{(n-w)!} (n+\rho)^{-\alpha_0} (n-1+\rho)^{-\alpha_1} (n-2+\rho)^{-\alpha_2}. \quad (6.87)$$

For Eq. (6.87) I used $n = 5$, $w = 2$, $a = 1$, $\alpha_0 = \alpha_1 = 1$ and $\alpha_2 = 3$. To calculate P_2, probabilities for all paths have to be added. Here, fortunately, we only

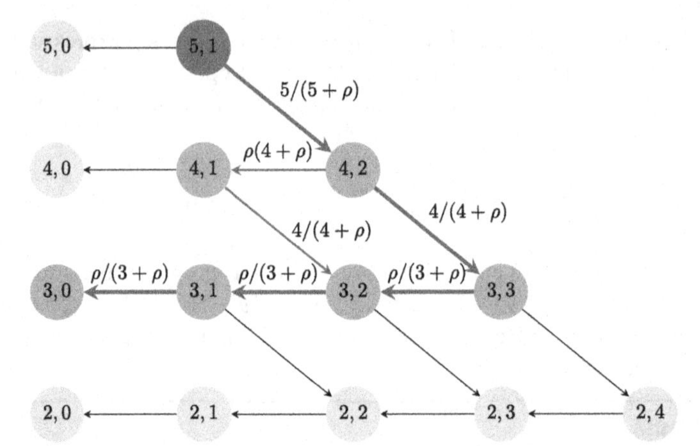

Figure 6.1 Possible paths (labeled edges—shown in red in online figure) from the start of the outbreak ($n = 5, a = 1$) to a final size of 2 (not counting the index case). The bottom two rows of the graph ($r = 1$ and $r = 0$) are omitted. The dark gray (bright red in online figure) node (5, 1) marks the start of the outbreak. Only nodes marked by a medium or dark gray (red in online figure) disk are relevant for the final outcome (3, 0).

have to deal with one alternative path (marked by edge shown as thin red line in online Fig. 6.1), $(5, 1) \to (4, 2) \to (4, 1) \to (3, 2) \to (3, 0)$. The corresponding probability is $P_{2,2} : \alpha_0 = 1, \alpha_1 = 2, \alpha_w = 2$.

Accordingly, the general formula for P_w given $w = 2, n = 5, a = 1$ is

$$P_w = \frac{\rho^{w+a} n!}{(n-w)!} \sum_{\alpha_0,\alpha_1,\alpha_2} (n+\rho)^{-\alpha_0}(n-1+\rho)^{-\alpha_1}(n-2+\rho)^{-\alpha_w} \tag{6.88}$$

for $(\alpha_0, \alpha_1, \alpha_w) \in [(1, 1, 3), (1, 2, 2)]$, i.e. the values of the αs are two constellations we have seen for the two paths. The expressions for $P_0, \ldots, P_5$ are written down in Bailey's Table 2. Note the discrepancy with Eq. (6.83).

By plugging-in numbers, the results from Bailey's Table 2 that lists final size calculations of outbreaks in very small populations (= household outbreaks) can be verified, for example, for $n = 5$, P_2. In this example, the term $(2\rho + 7)$ is the result of transforming the sum of fractions so that their denominators are their least common denominator, here $\frac{1}{(\rho+5)\,(\rho+4)^2\,(\rho+3)^3}$. The same is true for the complicated polynomials in the expressions for P_3, P_4, etc.

The reason why I went to great length to go through Bailey's discussion of Foster's formula is, however, Bailey's introduction of the estimation of transmission parameters using *maximum likelihood estimation* from data. I will not get much into the vast statistical theory of maximum likelihood estimation, but will merely outline the fundamentals. If we have expressions for P_w for $w \in \{0, 1, \ldots, n\}$, we can write out the likelihood which is defined as for our case as

$$\mathcal{L}(\rho|x) = \prod_{w=0}^{n} P_w^{a_w} \tag{6.89}$$

where a_w is the number of outbreaks with w infecteds. Given that expressions for P_w are quite "messy" (see Bailey's Table 2), the full likelihood becomes barely manageable. Usually, to find the maximum likelihood estimate, the natural logarithm of the likelihood, the *log-likelihood function* is maximized with respect to the parameter of interest. This is accomplished by setting the first derivative of the log-likelihood—referred to by Bailey as *score*—to zero and solving for the parameter, here ρ. The natural logarithm of the likelihood is used instead of the likelihood because the product (6.89) is thus transformed into a sum which is much easier to differentiate while leaving the location of the maximum unchanged. The first derivative of the log-likelihood can be found using the chain rule and the fact that the derivative of $\log(f(x))$ with respect to x is

$$\frac{d\log(f(x))}{dx} = \frac{df(x)}{dx}\frac{1}{f(x)}.$$

This equation may not be solvable analytically, but a numerical solution can often be found, e.g. by using the Newton–Raphson algorithm or similar methods.

Question 6.q

What does ρ represent? What about the transmission parameter?

6.5 P. Whittle: Comment on Bailey

6.5.1 Introduction

The last paper we will scrutinize in this chapter was published by Whittle under the title "The outcome of a stochastic epidemic—a note on Bailey's paper" [9]. It is, like suggested by the title, a direct response to Bailey's second paper [2] which we discussed in the previous section. Whittle states in the abstract that

> *"[...] the probability distribution (P_w) of the ultimate number of infected individuals (w) may be calculated by solving a certain set of doubly recurrent relations. I propose to show that for quite a general case these same probabilities may be obtained by the solution of a set of singly recurrent relation."*

Question 6.r

Referring to the quote, what could Whittle mean by *doubly recurrent relations*?

Whittle then formulates the following partial differential equation of p_{rs} with respect to t:

$$\frac{\partial p_{rs}}{\partial t} = A_{r+1}(s-1)p_{r+1,s-1} + B(s+1)p_{r,s+1} - (A_r s + Bs)p_{rs} \tag{6.90}$$

where B represents the removal rate (per infectious) and A_r the infection rate (per infectious individual) in r susceptibles. Whittle does not assume a particular functional form of A_r. In contrast to Bailey, Whittle does not scale time (i.e. divide) by the transmission parameter, and therefore both parameters show up in the equations.

Taking the Laplace transform of this equation, the following is obtained:

$$(\lambda + A_r s + Bs)q_{rs} = A_{r+1}(s-1)q_{r+l,s-1} + B(s+1)q_{r,s+l} + \delta_{nr}\delta_{as}. \tag{6.91}$$

The term $\delta_{nr}\delta_{as}$ is the product of two *Kronecker Delta* functions. The Kronecker Delta is defined as

$$\delta_{ij} = \begin{cases} 1, & \text{if } i = j, \\ 0, & \text{otherwise.} \end{cases} \tag{6.92}$$

Accordingly, $\delta_{nr} = 1$ if (and only if) $r = n$, i.e. if no individuals have become infected yet by the index case, and $\delta_{as} = 1$ if $s = a$, i.e. if the number of infecteds equals the number of index cases a. The product of the two can *only* be 1 if nobody has become infected yet *and* the index case has not recovered yet—in other words, nothing has happened epidemiologically, yet. Otherwise, $\delta_{nr}\delta_{as} = 0$.

Question 6.s

Derive the Laplace transform (6.91) of (6.90).

Referring to Bailey [2], Eq. (6.74) is written as

$$P_w = Bf_{n-w,1} \tag{6.93}$$

where Bailey's ρ is replaced here by Whittle's B. As before, $f_{rs} = \lim_{\lambda \to 0} q_{rs}$ and, therefore, $f_{n-w,1} = \lim_{\lambda \to 0} q_{n-w,1}$.

6.5.2 Recurrence relationship

Let

$$h_{r0} = 0, \tag{6.94}$$
$$h_{rs} = sf_{rs} \tag{6.95}$$

for $s = 1, 2, \ldots$. Eq. (6.91) can thus be written in terms of h_{rs} by letting λ go to zero and by replacing $(s-1)f_{r+1,s-1}$ by $h_{r+1,s-1}$, etc.:

$$(A_r + B)h_{rs} = A_{r+1}h_{r+l,s-1} + Bh_{r,s+l}, \tag{6.96}$$
$$(A_n + B)h_{ns} = Bh_{n,s+l} + \delta_{as}. \tag{6.97}$$

By dividing both sides of these equations by $(A_r + b)$ and $(A_n + B)$, respectively, we obtain

$$h_{rs} = \frac{B}{A_{r+1}} h_{r,s+l} \frac{A_{r+1}}{(A_r + B)} h_{r+l,s-1}, \tag{6.98}$$

$$h_{ns} = \frac{B}{(A_n + B)} h_{n,s+l} + \frac{\delta_{as}}{(A_n + B)}. \tag{6.99}$$

Whittle does not show these intermediate steps (Eqs. (6.96), (6.97), (6.98), and (6.99)), but proceeds to define

$$\alpha_r = \frac{B}{A_r + B}, \tag{6.100}$$

$$\beta_r = \frac{A_{r+1}}{A_r + B}. \tag{6.101}$$

Eqs. (6.98) and (6.99) can thus be written as

$$h_{rs} = \alpha_r h_{r,s+l} + \beta_r h_{r+l,s-1}, \tag{6.102}$$

$$h_{ns} = \alpha_n h_{n,s+l} + \beta_n \frac{\delta_{as}}{(A_{n+1})}. \tag{6.103}$$

The second term of the right-hand side of Eq. (6.103) is derived from

$$\begin{aligned} \frac{\delta_{as}}{(A_n + B)} &= \frac{1}{(A_n + B)} \frac{\delta_{as}}{1} \\ &= \frac{A_{n+1}}{(A_n + B)} \frac{\delta_{as}}{A_{n+1}} \text{ (multiply by } 1 = \frac{A_{n+1}}{A_{n+1}}) \\ &= \beta_n \frac{\delta_{as}}{A_{n+1}} \text{ (using Eq. (6.101), } \frac{A_{n+1}}{A_n + B} = \beta_n). \end{aligned}$$

Whittle then uses an ingenious "trick" to transform the *double* recurrence relationship into a *simple* recurrence one, by making the s "disappear" using the definition

$$H_r(x) = \sum_{s=1}^{\infty} h_{rs} x^{s+1}. \tag{6.104}$$

Note that $H_r(x)$ represents the generating function $A(x) = \sum_{n=0}^{\infty} a_n x^n = a_0 + a_1 x + a_2 x^2 + a_3 x^3 + \cdots$ modified in the following way—in our case, $a_n = h_{rn}$:

1. $a_0 = h_{r0}$ subtracted from $A(x)$ to obtain $A(x) - h_{r0} = h_{r1}x + h_{r2}x^2 + h_{r3}x^3 + \cdots$.
2. Then $A(x) - h_{r0}$ is multiplied by x to get $(A(x) - h_{r0})\ x = h_{r1}x^2 + h_{r2}x^3 + h_{r3}x^4 + \cdots$.

Generating functions can be powerful tools with many applications. For an introduction, see, for example, [10].

If Eq. (6.102) is multiplied by x^{s+1} and summed over s, the following can be obtained:

$$H_r(x) = \frac{x^2}{x - \alpha_r} \left[\beta_r H_{r+1}(x) - \alpha_r h_{r1} \right] \text{ (Whittle's Eq. (12)).} \tag{6.105}$$

Question 6.t

Derive Eq. (6.105).

Whittle continues

"A direct solution of (9) [our (6.102)] shows that

$$h_{r1} = \frac{\beta_r}{\alpha_r} H_{r+1}(\alpha_r), \tag{6.106}$$

as, indeed, it must, if the expression (12) [our (6.105)] for H_r is to constitute a finite series in x." (p. 117)

What Whittle means by "direct solution" is this: Eq. (6.105) has to be solved recursively, starting at the top, i.e. the highest possible value of s and working our way down to $s = 1$. We know that s cannot be higher than $n + a - r$ (the a for the initially infectious). Whenever the sum of subscripts of h_{rs}, representing the numbers susceptible and the numbers infectious, exceeds $n + a$ the corresponding $h_{rs} = 0$. We therefore start with:

1. $h_{r,n+a-r} = \beta_r h_{r+1,n+a-r-1}$; note that the term $\alpha_r h_{r,n}$ is not defined (sum of subscripts of h too large!) and therefore does not contribute.
2. Furthermore,

$$\begin{aligned} h_{r,n+a-r-1} &= \alpha_r h_{r,n+a-r} + \beta_r h_{r+l,n+a-r-2} \\ &= \alpha_r \left(\beta_r h_{r+1,n+a-r-1}\right) + \beta_r h_{r+1,n+a-r-2} \\ &= \beta_r \left(\alpha_r^2 h_{r+1,n+a-r-1} + \alpha_r h_{r+1,n+a-r-2}\right). \end{aligned}$$

   Here, we simply replaced $h_{r,n+a-r}$ from the first line with the expression we obtained in the first step ($\beta_r h_{r+1,n+a-r-1}$).
3. Proceeding similarly for the next step, we obtain

$$h_{r,n+a-r-2} = \beta_r \left(\alpha_r^3 h_{r+1,n+a-r-1} + \alpha_r^2 h_{r+l,n+a-r-2} + \alpha_r h_{r+l,n+a-r-3}\right).$$

4. This can be continued until we arrive at h_{r1}. As the careful examination of the pattern reveals this will be achieved in a total of $n+a-r-1$ steps. In each step, except for the first one, our expression picks up an exponent in the α_r. The first term, the one that goes back to the first step, therefore will be $\alpha_r^{n+a-r-1} h_{r+1,n+a-r-1} = h_{r+1,n+a-r-1}\alpha_r^{n+a-r-1}$. The sum will consist of terms like $h_{rs}\alpha_r^s$, i.e. the whole sum will be

$$h_{r1} = \beta_r \sum_{s=1}^{n+a-r} h_{r+1,s}\alpha_r^s. \tag{6.107}$$

   As the highest subscript corresponding to s defined is $n + a - r$ (the others are just 0), we could equivalently write $\sum_{s=1}^{\infty} h_{r+1,s}\alpha_r^s$.

5. Multiplying Eq. (6.107) by α_r, we get

$$\begin{aligned}
\alpha_r h_{r1} &= \alpha_r \beta_r \sum_{s=1}^{\infty} h_{r+1,s}\alpha_r^s \\
&= \beta_r \sum_{s=1}^{\infty} h_{r+1,s}\alpha_r^{s+1} \text{ (because } \alpha_r \times \alpha_r^s = \alpha_r^{s+1}) \\
\alpha_r h_{r1} &= \beta_r H_{r+1}(\alpha_r) \text{ (using Eq. (6.104) to replace} \qquad (6.108) \\
&\quad \sum_{s=1}^{\infty} h_{r+1,s} \text{ with } H_{r+1}(\alpha_r)) \\
h_{r1} &= \frac{\beta_r}{\alpha_r} H_{r+1}(\alpha_r) \text{ (divide by } \alpha_r). \qquad (6.109)
\end{aligned}$$

This last equation (6.109) is the required result (6.106).

This expression (6.106) for h_{rs} can now be used in Eq. (6.105) to give Whittle's Eq. (14) which is key:

$$\begin{aligned}
H_r(x) &= \frac{x^2}{x-\alpha_r}\left[\beta_r H_{r+1}(x) - \alpha_r h_{r1}\right] \\
&= \frac{x^2}{x-\alpha_r}\left[\beta_r H_{r+1}(x) - \alpha_r \frac{\beta_r}{\alpha_r} H_{r+1}(\alpha_r)\right], \\
H_r(x) &= \frac{\beta_r x^2}{x-\alpha_r}\left[H_{r+1}(x) - H_{r+1}(\alpha_r)\right] \text{ (factoring } \beta_r). \qquad (6.110)
\end{aligned}$$

This clearly represents a singly-recurrent equation for $H_r(x)$ as only one index/subscript is involved—r represents the number susceptible. There is, however, as Whittle points out, a difficulty with the fact that this expression does not seem to hold for $r = n$ as that would depend on H_{r+1}, but Whittle introduces the function

$$H_{n+1}(x) = \frac{x^a}{A_{n+1}}, \qquad (6.111)$$

only referring to Eq. (6.103) (Whittle's (9)). Eq. (6.111) can be derived as follows:

1. Derive the expression for h_{n1} using Eq. (6.111), starting with h_{na}:

a. $h_{na} = \beta_n \frac{1}{A_{n+1}}$; note that the first term of Eq. (6.111) vanishes because $h_{n,a+1}$ is not defined. The numerator of the fraction derives from δ_{as} which equals one as, here, $a = s$.

b. Also

$$\begin{aligned}
h_{n,a-1} &= \alpha_n h_{n,a} \text{ (} \beta_n \frac{\delta_{as}}{A_{n+1}} \text{ vanishes because } s \neq a) \\
&= \beta_n \frac{\alpha_n}{A_{n+1}}.
\end{aligned}$$

Finally, we can use Eqs. (6.93), (6.95), and (6.106) to proceed as follows:

1. We have $P_w = Bf_{n-w,1}$ (6.93).
2. Rearranging Eq. (6.95), we can write $f_{n-w,s} = \frac{h_{n-w,s}}{s}$ or $f_{n-w,1} = \frac{h_{n-w,1}}{1} = h_{n-w,1}$, yielding $P_w = Bh_{n-w,1}$.
3. Replacing $h_{n-w,1}$ with the expression suggested by Eq. (6.106), namely $h_{n-w,1} = \frac{\beta_r}{\alpha_r} H_{r+1}(\alpha_r)$, we obtain

$$P_w = B\frac{\beta_{n-w}}{\alpha_{n-w}} H_{n-w+1}(\alpha_{n-w}). \tag{6.112}$$

With Eq. (6.112) (Whittle's Eq. (16)) Whittle has achieved his most important goal: To quantify the probability distribution of the outcomes of this stochastic epidemic based on a—singly—recurrent relationship.

Question 6.u

How would you go about to calculating the probabilities of a particular epidemiologic outcome?

Whittle then introduces, without much of an explanation, his Eq. (17),

$$\begin{aligned}\sum_{w=0}^{u} \kappa_{n-u+1,n-u}\kappa_{n-u+2,n-u}\cdots\kappa_{n_w,n-u}\frac{\beta_{n-w}}{\alpha_{n-w}}P_w \\ = \kappa_{n-u+1,n-u}\kappa_{n-u+2,n-u}\cdots\kappa_{n,n-u}\left(\frac{B}{A_{n+1}}\right)\alpha_{n-u}^{a}\end{aligned} \tag{6.113}$$

with $\kappa_{rr} = 1$ and $\kappa_{rs} = \frac{\alpha_s^2\beta_r}{\alpha_s-\alpha_r}$, and states

"The final relation of (17), for u = n, reduces to

$$\sum_{0}^{n} P_w = 1,$$

provided that A_0 is zero, as it must be." (bottom of p. 117)

Question 6.v

Why is $A_0 = 0$, "as it must be"?

To understand Eq. (6.113), we can resort to the answer to Question 6.u and use Eqs. (6.157) and (6.112) to recursively compute P_w with w increasing. The definition of κ_{rs} will simplify the handling of the equations. We have to compute $H_r(x)$ recursively as we did for $H_{10}(x)$ until we arrive at $H_{n-w+1}(x)$ if we want to compute P_w:

1. We have already the expression for

$$\begin{aligned} H_{10}(x) &= \frac{\beta_{10}x^2}{x-\alpha_{10}}\left[\frac{x}{A_{n+1}} - P_0\frac{\alpha_{10}}{\beta_{10}}\frac{1}{B}\right] \\ &= \kappa_{10,x}\left[\frac{x}{A_{11}} - P_0\frac{\alpha_{10}}{\beta_{10}}\frac{1}{B}\right] \end{aligned} \tag{6.114}$$

and from this we calculate P_1,

$$P_1 = B\frac{\beta_9}{\alpha_9}\kappa_{10,9}\left[\frac{\alpha_9}{A_{11}} - P_0\frac{\alpha_{10}}{\beta_{10}}\frac{1}{B}\right].$$

2. This we can use to get $H_9(x)$:

$$\begin{aligned} H_9(x) &= \kappa_{9,x}\left[H_{10}(\alpha_x) - P_1\frac{\alpha_9}{\beta_9}\frac{1}{B}\right] \\ &= \kappa_{9,x}\left[\kappa_{10,x}\left[\frac{\alpha_x}{A_{11}} - P_0\frac{\alpha_{10}}{\beta_{10}}\frac{1}{B}\right] - P_1\frac{\alpha_9}{\beta_9}\frac{1}{B}\right]. \end{aligned} \tag{6.115}$$

3. Eq. (6.156), in combination with Eq. (6.112), is used to calculate P_2:

$$\begin{aligned} P_2 &= B\frac{\beta_8}{\alpha_8}H_9(\alpha_8) \\ &= B\frac{\beta_8}{\alpha_8}\kappa_{9,8}\left[\kappa_{10,8}\left[\frac{\alpha_8}{A_{11}} - P_0\frac{\alpha_{10}}{\beta_{10}}\frac{1}{B}\right] - P_1\frac{\alpha_9}{\beta_9}\frac{1}{B}\right]. \end{aligned} \tag{6.116}$$

After multiplying out the right-hand side of (6.116) and bringing all P_1 and P_0 over to the left-hand side, we obtain:

$$P_2 + B\frac{\beta_8}{\alpha_8}\frac{\alpha_9}{\beta_9}\frac{1}{B}\kappa_{9,8}P_1 + B\frac{\beta_8}{\alpha_8}\frac{\alpha_{10}}{\beta_{10}}\frac{1}{B}\kappa_{9,8}\kappa_{10,8}P_0 = B\frac{\beta_8}{\alpha_8}\frac{\alpha_8}{A_{11}}\kappa_{9,8}\kappa_{10,8}, \tag{6.117}$$

$$\frac{\alpha_8}{\beta_8}P_2 + \kappa_{9,8}\frac{\alpha_9}{\beta_9}P_1 + \kappa_{9,8}\kappa_{10,8}\frac{\alpha_{10}}{\beta_{10}}P_0 = \kappa_{9,8}\kappa_{10,8}\left(\frac{B}{A_{11}}\right)\alpha_8, \tag{6.118}$$

$$\sum_{w=0}^{2}\left(\prod_{v=0}^{w}\kappa_{8+v,8}\right)\frac{\alpha_{10-w}}{\beta_{10-w}}P_w = \left(\prod_{v=1}^{u}\kappa_{8+v,8}\right)\left(\frac{B}{A_{11}}\right)\alpha_8, \tag{6.119}$$

$$\sum_{w=0}^{u}\left(\prod_{v=0}^{w}\kappa_{n-u+v,n-u}\right)\frac{\alpha_{n-w}}{\beta_{n-w}}P_w = \left(\prod_{v=1}^{u}\kappa_{n-u+v,n-u}\right)\cdot\left(\frac{B}{A_{n+1}}\right)\alpha_{n-u}. \tag{6.120}$$

A few explanations on Eqs. (6.117) through (6.120): First, we divided both sides of Eq. (6.117) by $\frac{\beta_8}{\alpha_8}$ and rearranged the left-hand side. I then displayed the product of the κ_{rs} using the product symbol. Finally, I used symbols for u and v to make the similarity with expression (6.113) more obvious.

Using a small number for n it can be, more or less easily, verified that, in fact, $\sum_{w=0}^{n} P_w = 1$.

6.5.3 A slow wind-down—not without somewhat of a(n anti-)climax

Whittle points out (top of p. 118) that at the initial stages of an epidemic in a large population the number of susceptibles changes very little from a transmission event to a transmission event. This is true because one—which is the number by which the susceptibles decrease after one transmission event—may be vanishingly small compared to the whole population n. Therefore, for $A_r \approx A_t$. Equivalently, $A_r - A_t \approx 0$.

For the sake of the argument, we even assume that, for any r, $A_r = A$, i.e. the transmission parameter is constant. Accordingly, $\alpha_r = \alpha$ because $\alpha = \frac{B}{A+B}$.

This has the, somewhat unpleasant, consequence that expression (6.113) is no longer defined because $\kappa_{rs} = \frac{\alpha^2\beta}{\alpha-\alpha} = \frac{\alpha^2\beta}{0}$ (division by 0).

However, the problem can be solved as follows: Let us first consider $H_n(x)$ plugging-in n for r in (6.110):

$$H_n(x) = \frac{\beta_n x^2}{x - \alpha_n}\left[H_{n+1}(x) - H_{n+1}(\alpha_n)\right].$$

If we substitute the right-hand side of (6.111) for H_{n+1}, this becomes

$$\begin{aligned} H_n(x) &= \frac{\beta_n x^2}{x - \alpha_n^a}\left[\frac{x^a}{A_{n+1}} - \frac{\alpha_n^a}{A_{n+1}}\right] \\ &= \frac{\frac{\beta_n x^2}{A_{n+1}}\left(x^a - \alpha_n^a\right)}{x - \alpha_n}. \end{aligned} \tag{6.121}$$

Rearranging expression (6.121) and letting x go to α_n, we obtain

$$\lim_{x\to\alpha_n} H_n(x) = \frac{\beta_n x^2 \left(x^a - \alpha_n^a\right)}{A_{n+1}\,(x - \alpha_n)}. \tag{6.122}$$

Clearly, when $x \to \alpha_n$ the numerator and denominator will both vanish. This situation is conveniently addressed by the famous L'Hôpital's rule that states that, if the limit of the numerator and denominator of a ratio, which are both zero or both infinity, is considered then the limit of the ratio equals the limit of the ratio of the derivatives (this is casually stated). Whittle uses that to do address this problem: Differentiating both the numerator and denominator of (6.122), the following is obtained:

$$\begin{aligned} \lim_{x\to\alpha} \frac{\beta_n x^2 \left(x^a - \alpha_n^a\right)}{A_{n+1}\,(x - \alpha_n)} &= \lim_{x\to\alpha_n} \frac{\beta_n x^{2+a} - \beta_n x^2 \alpha_n^a}{A_{n+1}\,(x - \alpha_n)} \\ &= \lim_{x\to\alpha_n} \frac{(2+a)\,\beta_n x^{2+a-1} - 2\,\beta_n x\,\alpha_n^a}{A_{n+1}} \\ &= \frac{(2+a)\,\beta_n\,\alpha_n^{a+1} - 2\,\beta_n \alpha_n^{a+1}}{A_{n+1}} \\ &\quad \text{(differentiating with respect to } x\text{)} \\ &= \frac{a\,\beta_n\,\alpha_n^{a+1}}{A_{n+1}} \text{ (simplifying the difference in numerator)} \end{aligned}$$

$$= \frac{a\ A_{n+1}\ B^{a+1}}{(A_n + B)^{a+2}\ A_{n+1}}$$

(expressing α_n and β in terms of A_{10} and B)

$$= \frac{a\ B^{a+1}}{(A_n + B)^{a+2}}. \quad (6.123)$$

To compute P_1 from that, Eq. (6.123) could then be plugged-in into (6.112):

$$\begin{aligned} P_1 &= B\,\frac{\beta_n}{\alpha_n}\,H_n(\alpha_n) \\ &= \frac{a\ A_{n+1}\ B^{a+1}}{(A_n + B)^{a+2}}\ \text{(simplifying fraction } \frac{\beta_n}{\alpha_n} \text{ yields } \frac{A_{n+1}}{B}\text{)}. \end{aligned}$$

This—almost—precisely corresponds to Whittle's Eq. (21) (top of p. 118):

$$\left.\begin{aligned} P_w &= \frac{A^w B^{a+w}}{(A+B)^{a+2w}}\,\frac{a(a+2w-1)!}{w!(a+w)!} \\ P_n &= 1 - \sum_{w=0}^{n-1} P_w \end{aligned}\right\} \quad (w = 0, 1, \ldots, n-1) \quad (6.124)$$

and provides a means to approximately compute P_w for low w if the population (n) is large. Do you see why I said "almost"? The subscripts in the As of Whittle's Eq. (21) have been, rightfully, dropped as in each step the identity of α_r and α_{r+1} (and thus of A_r and A_{r+1}) is ensured.

Question 6.w

Assume that $n = 5$, $A_r = 0.1 \times r$ and $B = 0.3$. Calculate P_0, i.e. the probability of no secondary infections using first Bailey's then Whittle's methods.

Whittle concludes this section with a brief discussion of the common assumption that $A_r = C\,r$, i.e. that the transmission hazard is proportional to the number of susceptibles available. I will not discuss this part.

The last section of Whittle's paper, entitled "3. The Probability of Epidemic" is, in some sense, pivotal to not only this paper, but even to this whole discussion of stochastic transmission models as the implied question is so crucial: "Is, under given circumstances, a true epidemic possible?" Obviously, the answer to that question has enormous public health implications; furthermore, it is also of great theoretical merit.

Whittle begins with the following definition (top of p. 119):

> *"It shall be said that an epidemic has (has not) taken place if the total proportion of susceptibles which become infected exceeds (does not exceed) a predetermined fraction γ. With this definition the probability of no epidemic is*
>
> $$\pi_\gamma = \sum_{w=0}^{n\gamma} P_w, \quad (6.125)$$
>
> *where P_w is in general given by (17) [our Eq. (6.113)]."*

The quantity π_γ thus represents the probability that not more than a proportion γ of the population becomes infected during the course of the outbreak or the probability of no epidemic, given the criterion γ which corresponds to $n\,\gamma$ individuals infected at most.

For once, possibly to the delight of the reader, I am skipping details here, because I myself was unable to replicate some of the steps.[2]

Instead, I will give a summary here:

- Two alternative "models" of the transmission hazard A are assumed: One that is lower than A, $A_{n(1-y)}$, and one that is higher, A_n–all are constants. The corresponding probabilities of no epidemic, π, are ordered correspondingly: The higher the infection hazard A the lower the associated π.
- Whittle then presents the equation

$$\sum_{w=0}^{n\gamma} S_w(A) = \sum_{w=0}^{\infty} S_w(A) - R_{n\gamma}(A), \tag{6.126}$$

  where $S_w(A)$ is nothing but the P_w from Eq. (6.124) and $R_{n\gamma}(A) = \sum_{w=n\gamma+1}^{\infty}$. He shows that $R_{n\gamma}(A)$ becomes negligible for large n; thus that term will be neglected.
- Without further explanation he presents the equality

$$\sum_{w=0}^{\infty} = \left[\frac{A+B-|A-B|}{2A}\right]^a. \tag{6.127}$$

- Eq. (6.127) is then used with A_n and $A_{n(1-\gamma)}$ to the probabilities of no epidemic, the complement of which is the *probability of an epidemic*.
- Using instead of A_n and B he then uses Bailey's removal parameter $\rho_n = nB/A_n$ to come to the climactic statement:

$$\left.\begin{array}{l}\text{For } \rho_n < n \text{ the probability of epidemic is } 1-(\rho_n/n)^a.\\ \text{For } \rho_n > n \text{ the probability of epidemic is zero.}\end{array}\right\} \tag{6.128}$$

This is the stochastic equivalent to Kermack & McKendrick's threshold theorem and in opposition to Bailey's statement to the contrary (p. 132). Why, in the title of this section, I also referred to an "anti-climatic" aspect is the obscurity of the argument which may, in fact, be absolutely sound. Furthermore, the derivation of (6.128) is based on the assumption of an constant A, which may be justified for the early stages of an outbreak in a large population when the numbers of susceptibles, relative to n barely decline, but which may not be a meaningful approximation when all possible trajectories of the outbreak are considered.

[2] I cannot exclude the possibility of typographical errors. For example, in Whittle's Eq. (24), which I did not further discuss, α_{n-u}^{u-w} is misspelled as α_{n-u}^{-w}.

Appendix 6.A Answers

6.a There is no clear right answer to this question. One possible reason is the fact that ordinary differential equations, especially since the advent of easy-accessible computational power, are easier to work with than stochastic models that require a different set of mathematical skills. Also, stochastic models rapidly become prohibitively complex.

6.b Eq. (6.10) is a closed-form solution for the number susceptible as a function of time. This is an exceptional case as most differential equations encountered in transmission models cannot be analytically solved. They can, however, always be numerically solved, by the use of various algorithms (Euler method, Runge–Kutta method, etc.).

6.c The word *number* was set in quotes because, as pointed out elsewhere in this book, ordinary differential equation transmission models treat the susceptible, infectious and recovered as *quantities* that vary continuously. This can be a poor representation of transmission phenomena, especially if the numbers are small.

6.d These rates are driven by the numbers of susceptibles and infectious individuals as well as by a transmission coefficient which captures both the contact process and the probability of transmitting the infectious agent in question (see, e.g. Chap. 4). If there are r susceptibles there are $(n - r + 1)$ infectious individuals; remember that the $+1$ is due to the "single infectious individual which is introduced into the population" [1, p. 194]. So we would get a rate of $r(n - r + 1)$—but what happened to the transmission coefficient? As I explained on p. 109 of this chapter, the transmission coefficient is "integrated" in the time measure and we *should* write t^* instead of t. When first encountered, this may be difficult to grasp. But what that means is that, say, one day measured on the scale of t is one, while measured on the scale of t^* is $1 \times \beta$. Assuming a value of $\beta = 0.1$, one day would be $t^* = 1 \times \beta = 0.1$. Vice versa, $t^* = 1$ corresponds to $t = 1/\beta = 10$—confusing!

6.e We first have to take the Laplace transform of $\frac{dp_r(t)}{dt}$:

$$\int_0^\infty e^{-\lambda t} \frac{dp_r(t)}{dt} dt = \int_0^\infty e^{-\lambda t} dp_r(t) \tag{6.129}$$

$$= e^{-\lambda t} p_r(t)\Big|_0^\infty + \lambda \int_0^\infty e^{-\lambda t} p_r(t) dt \tag{6.130}$$

$$= \lambda q_r \tag{6.131}$$

where q_r is the Laplace transform of $p_r(t)$. Some further explanations:

- Eq. (6.129): (Right-hand side) This is simply the application of the Laplace transform (6.13) to $\frac{dp_r(t)}{dt}$; (left-hand side) dt in the derivative and in the integral cancel.
- Eq. (6.130): Integration-by-parts is performed on $\int_0^\infty e^{-\lambda t} dp_r(t)$: $\int u dv = uv - \int v du$, where $u = e^{-\lambda t}$ and $\frac{du}{dt} = -\lambda e^{-\lambda t}$; multiplying $\frac{du}{dt}$ by dt renders $du = -\lambda e^{-\lambda t} dt$. Similarly, $dv = dp_r(t)$ and $v = \int dp_r(t) = p_r(t)$. The expression uv

in the general integration-by-parts formula becomes $e^{-\lambda t} p_r(t)\big|_0^\infty$ because we are dealing with a definite, although improper (limit ∞) integral.
- Eq. (6.130), first term on the right-hand side:

$$\begin{aligned} e^{-\lambda t} p_r(t)\big|_0^\infty &= \lim_{t\to\infty} e^{-\lambda t} p_r(t) - e^{-\lambda 0} p_r(0) \\ &= 0 - 0. \end{aligned}$$

The first 0 is due to the fact that $\lim_{w\to\infty} e^{-\lambda w} = 0$; the second 0 results from the boundary conditions stated in the question, $p_r(0) = 0$ for $r < n$. The expression corresponding to $\int v du$ (general integration-by-parts formula) in Eq. (6.130) is $\int_0^\infty p_r(t)(-\lambda e^{-\lambda t})dt = -\lambda \int_0^\infty p_r(t)e^{-\lambda t}$ because the $-\lambda$ can be taken outside the integral (just a constant). But $\int_0^\infty p_r(t)e^{-\lambda t}dt$ is nothing else than the definition of q_r. Therefore, $\int_0^\infty p_r(t)(-\lambda e^{-\lambda t})dt = -\lambda q_r$. This is the second term ($\int v du$; note that by subtracting the negative expression we *add* the expression) of the right-hand side of the integration-by-parts formula.

As the first expression (uv) vanishes, we can write the result, the Laplace transform of $\frac{dp_r(t)}{dt}$, as

$$\int_0^\infty e^{-\lambda t} \frac{dp_r(t)}{dt} dt = \lambda q_r. \tag{6.132}$$

6.f Eq. (6.16), $q_r = \frac{(r+1)(n-r)q_{r+1}}{\lambda + r(n-r+1)}$, allows us to calculate q_r from q_{r+1}. As we know $q_n = \frac{1}{\lambda+n}$, we could work our way "backwards" from $r = n$ all the way to $r = 0$; this is a *recursive* strategy:

1. Start with $q_n = \frac{1}{\lambda+n}$.

2. Then

$$\begin{aligned} q_{n-1} &= \frac{(n-1+1)(n-(n-1))}{\lambda + (n-1)(n-(n-1)+1)} q_n \\ &= \frac{(n-1+1)\,(n-(n-1))}{\lambda + (n-1)\,(n-(n-1)+1)} \times \frac{1}{\lambda+n} \\ &= \frac{n\,1}{\lambda + (n-1)\,2} \times \frac{1}{\lambda+n}. \end{aligned}$$

Note that I have substituted $\frac{1}{\lambda+n}$ (first line) for $q_{n-1+1} = q_n$ (second line—see Eq. (6.19)).

3. Next,

$$q_{n-2} = \frac{(n-1)\,2}{\lambda + (n-2)\,3} \times \frac{n\,1}{\lambda + (n-1)\,2} \times \frac{1}{\lambda+n}.$$

Here, we have used the expression calculated for q_{n-1} and plugged that into the general recursive formula (Eq. (6.16)).

4. Then

$$q_{n-3} = \frac{(n-2)\,3}{\lambda + (n-3)\,4} \times \frac{(n-1)\,2}{\lambda + (n-2)\,3} \times \frac{n\,1}{\lambda + (n-1)\,2} \times \frac{1}{\lambda+n}.$$

So, for the general case we have

$$q_r = \frac{(r+1)(n-r)}{\lambda + r(n-r+1)} \times \frac{(r+2)(n-r-1)}{\lambda + (r+1)(n-r)} \times \cdots \times \frac{n\,1}{\lambda + (n-1)\,2} \times \frac{1}{\lambda + n}. \tag{6.133}$$

6.g The two random variables X (infectious) and Y (susceptible) can change at time t in the following ways:

1. If a susceptible becomes infected/infectious at time t, $X = x$ will increase by one, i.e. $x \to x+1$, while y will decrease by one, $y \to y-1$.
2. If an infectious individual recovers from infectiousness x will decline, i.e. $x \to x-1$, leaving y unchanged.

So assuming this simple "Kermack & McKendrick model", there are only two types of processes.

6.h The answer should become more apparent when the probability-generating function (6.32) is written in the following way:

$$\Pi(z, w, t) = \sum_{x,y} p(x, y, t)\, z^y w^x \tag{6.134}$$

$$= p(0,0,t)z^0w^0 + p(0,1,t)z^1w^0 + p(0,2,t)z^2w^0 + \cdots + p(N,0,t)z^0w^N \tag{6.135}$$

is written as in Eq. (6.134) above. But two comments first:

1. N, which would represent the whole population, is not really defined. As in the current transmission model, new susceptibles are recruited, but their number is not regulated, such that N could go to infinity and there would be an infinite sum. For the sake of simplicity, we therefore assume that N is fixed.
2. The (x, y) combination $(0, 0)$ is only possible if all susceptibles are exhausted and the last infectious is removed before a new susceptible is recruited.

So how can (6.134), or (6.135), change over time? Obviously, the terms $z^y w^x$, such as $z^{20} w^3$ are constant; the only thing that *can* change is the $p(x, y, t)$. For example, at $t = 0$, there is only the one index case (there could be more than one) and all the susceptibles. There hasn't been time to transmit anything yet, so $p(1, N, t = 0) = 1$ with all other $p(x, y, 0) = 0$. For any $t > 0$ all probabilities will be larger than 0 and smaller than 1. So, given that $z^y w^x$ are constant while the $p(x, y, t)$ change, we have the answer: (6.32) can change over time only *via* the probabilities.

6.i Just as for the first two terms, we first characterize the rate at which susceptible individuals are recruited and then quantify the resulting change with respect to the probability-generating function:

1. The rate at which susceptible individuals are recruited. This process, either based on immigration or reproduction is driven by the rate parameter ν (third row, middle column of Table 6.2). As the process is independent from both x and y, ν also equals the rate.

2. Adding of one susceptible individual results in *one more* susceptibles ($y + 1$). Accordingly, the term $z^y w^x$ of the probability-generating function is changed to $z^{y+1} w^x$. The *amount* of change in the probability-generating function due to new infection thus is

$$z^{y+1} w^x - z^y w^x. \tag{6.136}$$

3. The total amount of change in the probability-generating function at time t due to the recruitment of susceptible individuals if there are x infectious and y susceptible individuals is therefore given by the product of (6.34), ν and (6.136),

$$p(x, y) \times \nu \times \left(z^{y+1} w^x - z^y w^x\right). \tag{6.137}$$

Summing Eq. (6.137) over all values of x and y we get

$$\sum_{x,y} p(x, y) \times \nu \times \left(z^{y+1} w^x - z^y w^x\right). \tag{6.138}$$

Eq. (6.138) can be rearranged as follows:

$$\begin{aligned} \sum_{x,y} p(x, y)\nu \left(z^{y+1} w^x - z^y w^x\right) &= \sum_{x,y} p(x, y)\nu\,(w - 1)\, z^y w^x \\ &= \nu\,(w - 1) \sum_{x,y} p(x, y) z^y w^x \\ &= \nu\,(w - 1)\,\Pi \qquad (6.139) \\ &\quad \text{(noting that } \Pi = \sum_{x,y} p(x, y) z^y w^x\text{)} \end{aligned}$$

We have thus shown that the third term of the partial derivative of the probability-generating function with respect to time, i.e. the left-hand side of Eq. (6.33) captures the change in the probability-generating function over time that is due to recruitment of susceptible individuals.

6.j Let us first remind ourselves what that model really is:

1. At time $t = 0$ there are $y(0) = N$ susceptibles and one infectious (index case; $x(0) = 1$).
2. New infections arise at a rate $\lambda x(t) y(t)$.
3. Infectious individuals become infectious immediately after being infected.
4. Infectious individuals are "removed" at rate $\mu x(t)$, i.e. they become immune or die at this rate–note that, for this model, these very different outcomes are equivalent!
5. New susceptibles are added at a rate of ν.

As this is a stochastic model, these rates determine *random* transitions. There are many different ways of implementing this model. The only constant feature of these are pseudo-random numbers. Refer to the implementation of this model in R in the online supplement.

6.k Like we did for the first term of the right-hand side of Eq. (6.33), we will first take the partial derivatives of both terms with respect to w and then set both w and z

to one. The second term, $\mu(1-w)\frac{\partial \Pi}{\partial w}$ is, again, a function of two functions of w and can therefore be differentiated using the product rule:

$$\begin{aligned}\frac{\partial \mu(1-w)\frac{\partial \Pi}{\partial w}}{\partial w} &= \mu(1-w)\sum_{x,y} p(x,y)\,x(x-1)\,z^y w^{x-2} \\ &\quad -\mu\sum_{x} p(x)\,x\,z^y w^{x-1} &(6.140)\\ &= -\mu\sum_{x,y} p(x,y)\,x \\ &= -\mu E(X). &(6.141)\end{aligned}$$

Again, we applied the product rule to obtain the partial derivative of (6.46) with respect to w, (6.140). When setting $w = z = 1$, the first term of the sum on the right-hand side of (6.140) vanishes because $1 - w = 1 - 1 = 0$ and only $-\mu E(X)$ remains.
The third term, $\nu(z-1)\Pi$, can be dealt with accordingly:

$$\begin{aligned}\frac{\partial \nu(z-1)\Pi}{\partial w} &= \nu(z-1)\sum_{x,y} p(x,y)\,z^y w^x \\ &\quad +0\times\sum_{x,y} p(x,y)\,x\,z^y w^{x-1} \\ &= 0.\end{aligned}$$

The expression becomes 0 because for $z = 1$, $\nu(z-1) = 0$. Note that the partial derivative with respect to w is 0 even before setting $z \equiv 1$ because $\frac{\partial \nu(z-1)}{\partial w} = 0$ ($\nu(z-1)$ is, in terms of w, a constant and the derivative of a constant is 0).

6.l Bailey uses v instead of Bartlett's w and u instead of z and ρ for μ, but there also are two structural differences. The first one is where Bartlett, in the first expression of the right-hand side, multiplies the expression in parentheses by λ, the transmission parameter; there is no equivalent term in (6.57). This is due to the integration of λ or, rather, β (see [1], bottom of p. 194) into the time measure. I am not convinced that the slight simplification resulting from this "trick" is really worth the additional source of confusion. The second difference is due to the absence of "regeneration" in the "Kermack & McKendrick" model. The third term of Bartlett's partial differential equation is therefore missing.

6.m The recurrence relationship is given by Eqs. (6.65),

$$(r+1)(s-1)q_{r+1,s-1} - \{s(r+\rho)+\lambda\}q_{rs} + \rho(s+1)q_{r,s+1} = 0,$$

and (6.66),

$$-\{a(n+\rho)+\lambda\} = 0.$$

To derive the relationship, we have to revisit Eq. (6.59),

$$(v^2-uv)\frac{\partial^2\Pi^*}{\partial u\partial v} + \rho(1-v)\frac{\partial \Pi^*}{\partial v} - \lambda\Pi^* + u^n v^a = 0.$$

To equate the coefficients, we have to write out the different expressions above as sums:

1. $(v^2 - uv)\frac{\partial^2\Pi^*}{\partial u \partial v} = \sum_{r,s} rs\, q_{rs}\, u^{r-1} v^{s+1} - \sum_{r,s} rs\, q_{rs}\, u^r v^s$;
2. $\rho(1-v)\frac{\partial \Pi^*}{\partial v} = \sum_{r,s} \rho s\, q_{rs}\, u^r v^{s-1} - \sum_{r,s} \rho s\, q_{rs}\, u^r v^s$;
3. $-\lambda\Pi^* = -\lambda \sum_{r,s} q_{rs}\, u^r v^s$.

Now, we have to take the crucial step of collecting the $u^r v^s$, for example, all coefficients of $u^{10}v^5$, i.e. of all u that are to the power of 10 and v that are to the power of 5. To illustrate, I will continue with this example.

1. From the right-hand side of the first item above, we have:
   a. $11 \times 4\, u^{10} v^5\, q_{11,4}$, corresponding to $u^r v^s\, (r+1)(s-1)\, q_{r+1,s-1}$;
   b. $-10 \times 5\, u^{10} v^5\, q_{10,5}$, corresponding to $u^r v^s\, rs\, q_{rs}$.
   Note that the relationships between the exponents of u and v and the corresponding coefficients are determined by Eq. (6.59) which tells us how they relate. If, for example, the exponent of u is $r-1$ and the one of v is $s+1$ while the coefficient has an r and s (such as in q_{rs} or rs), we know that the values for r have to be larger by one (here 11) than the exponent of u (here 10) and the value of s (here 4) has to smaller by one than the exponent of v.
2. From the right-hand side of the second item above, we have:
   a. $\rho 6\, u^{10} v^5\, q_{10,6}$, corresponding to $\rho(s+1)\, u^r v^s\, q_{r,s+1}$;
   b. $-\rho 5\, u^{10} v^5\, q_{10,5}$, corresponding to $-\rho s\, u^r v^s\, q_{rs}$.
3. From the third item above, we have $-\lambda\, u^{10} v^5 q_{10,5}$.
4. The final summand, $u^n v^a$, only "counts" for $r = n, s = a$ (see below).

The coefficients of the above expressions can be combined and expressed, such that we have $u^r v^s$ instead of $u^{10}v^5$:

$q_{10,5}$: $-10 \times 5\, u^{10} v^5\, q_{10,5}$, $-\rho 5\, u^{10} v^5\, q_{10,5}$, and $-\lambda\, u^{10} v^5 q_{10,5}$ to give $q_{10,5}\, u^{10} v^5(-10 \times 5 - \rho 5 - \lambda)$. If we let $r = 10$ and $s = 5$ and thus $q_{rs} = q_{10,5}$, this can be expressed more generally as

$$-u^r v^s\, q_{rs}\, (s(r + \rho + \lambda)). \tag{6.142}$$

$q_{11,4}$: $11 \times 4\, u^{10} v^5\, q_{11,4}$, or

$$u^r v^s\, q_{r+1,s-1}\, (r+1)(s-1). \tag{6.143}$$

$q_{10,6}$: $\rho 6\, u^{10} v^5\, q_{10,6}$, or

$$u^r v^s\, q_{r,s+1}\, \rho\, (s+1)s. \tag{6.144}$$

Combining (6.142), (6.143), and (6.144):

$$\begin{aligned} 0 &= u^r v^s \left((r+1)(s-1)\, q_{r+1,s-1} - (s(r+\rho)+\lambda)\, q_{rs} + \rho\, s\, q_{r,s+1}\right), \\ 0 &= q_{r+1,s-1}\, (r+1)(s-1) - q_{rs}\, (s(r+\rho)+\lambda) + q_{r,s+1}\, \rho\, (s+1) \\ &\quad \text{(divide both sides by } u^r v^s\text{).} \end{aligned} \tag{6.145}$$

For the case $r = n, s = a$ this becomes

$$0 = q_{n+1,a-1}\, (n+1)(a-1) - q_{n,a}\, (a(n+\rho)+\lambda) + q_{n,a+1}\, \rho\, (a+1) + 1.$$

The 1 at the end of the expression derives from the $u^n v^a$ in (6.59) which we divide by $u^n v^a$. As there cannot be more than n susceptibles (no immigration or reproduction) and the number of susceptibles plus the number of infectious individuals cannot exceed $n+a$, this equation becomes

$$-q_{n,a}\,(a(n+\rho)+\lambda)+1=0. \tag{6.146}$$

Thus we have verified the recurrence relationship. Eq. (6.146) can be solved for $q_{n,a}$:

$$q_{n,a}=\frac{1}{a(n+\rho)+\lambda}. \tag{6.147}$$

6.n The answer to this question becomes obvious if we become clear about what we exactly mean by the "final size of an epidemic". The adjective *final* leaves little doubt that we are referring to the number of cases when nothing else happens, i.e. when no more cases arise. Given our model and our assumption, after the introduction of the initial cases, all cases result from transmission in the population we are modeling. Therefore, the epidemic will cease once the last infectious case is "removed". Accordingly, we are interested in all pairs (r,s) for which $s=0$; r can be anything between n and 0 which is the number of infections, not counting the index case(s). However, as $s=0$ is *always* preceded by $s=1$, i.e. when the last remaining infectious individual is removed, the pair $(r, 1)$ can also be considered relevant.

6.o Having expressions now for calculating P_w, we certainly have the means to calculate final size probabilities:

1. From Eq. (6.79) we first calculate $f_{5,1}$ (denoted by the red circle in Fig. 6.2, online version)—this is the only quantity that can be directly calculated from the parameters n, a, and ρ.
2. We can then use (6.74) to calculate $P_0=\rho f_{n,0}$; P_0 is the probability that there will be no outbreak at all! The empty circle (green border in online figure) alludes to the fact that this, like the other P_w, is the quantity of interest.
3. Having calculated $f_{n,1}=f_{5,1}$, we can calculate the first "diagonal" (shown as purple circles in Fig. 6.2, online version): these represent all the states that result from the initial infection, $r=n, s=1$, without any infectious being removed. The calculations are made in the order $f_{5,1}\to f_{4,2}$, $f_{4,2}\to f_{3,3},\ldots$. These calculations use the right-hand side of Eq. (6.80): $f_{rs}=(r+1)(s-1)f_{r+1,s-1}/(s(r+\rho))$; the second part of the numerator, $\rho(s+1)q_{n,s+1}$ is zero by definition because the number of susceptible and first part of the numerator of infectious would be larger than $n+1$ and thus not defined.
4. As the next step, $f_{4,1}$ is calculated from $f_{4,2}$ using the second part of the right-hand side of Eq. (6.80): $f_{rs}=(\rho(s+1)q_{r,s+1})/(s(r+\rho))$. $f_{4,1}$ is the "start" of the next "diagonal", calculating $f_{3,2}$, $f_{2,3}$, etc. using the full right-hand side of Eq. (6.80) because all these nodes have two edges leading to them.
5. The steps described in item **4.** are repeated until the diagonal $f_{1,1}\to f_{0,2}$ is reached.
6. From $f_{0,1},\ldots,f_{5,1}$ the corresponding probabilities $P_5,\ldots,P_0$ are calculated, using Eq. (6.74).

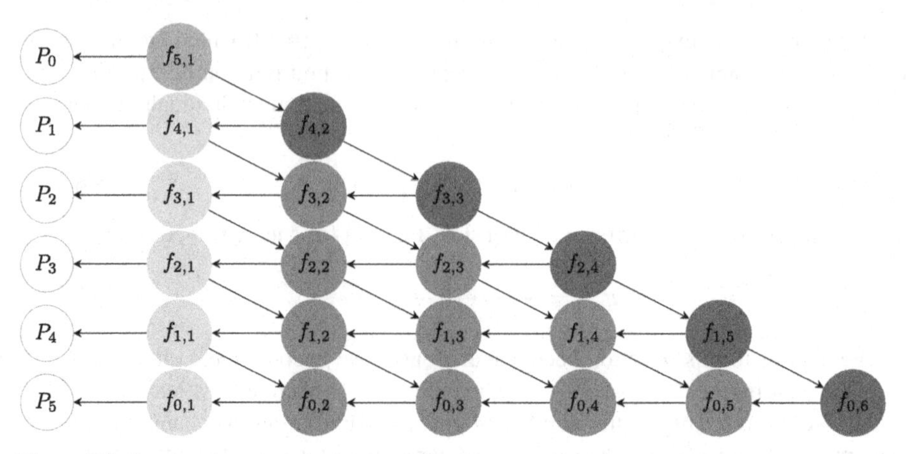

Figure 6.2 The recursive calculation of f_{rs}. See the answers to Questions 6.o & 6.p for explanations.

The algorithm is implemented using R (online supplement).

6.p $r/(r+\rho)$ and $\rho/(r+\rho)$ are *conditional* probabilities because they refer to the transitions from a particular state, defined by the number of susceptibles r. Interestingly, the number of infectious does not appear in these expressions. Why is that? Consider the rate of transitions from state r, s to $r-1, s+1$: This is clearly, as defined in the quote on page 127.

6.q While Bailey states that "the probability of one infected person being removed from circulation in time dt is $\rho y dt$" (see page 127) clearly suggests that ρ is the "removal parameter", this is, however, not quite true: Earlier in the paper he defines "$\rho = \gamma/\beta$, the ratio of the removal [γ] to infection rate [β]." This is due to the fact that he scales time by β. As Bailey points out:

> *"We cannot expect to be able to estimate β and γ separately as the asymptotic distribution of epidemic size for infinite time yields no information about the time scale. For this we should require data giving the time intervals between successive infections in families with two or more cases." (top of p. 184)*

This is an important and insightful statement which answers the second part of this question regarding β.

6.r *Doubly recurrent relations* refers to the fact that f_{rs} is calculated from $f_{r,s+1}$ and $f_{r+1,s-1}$. All the f_{rs} that require $f_{r,s+1}$ and $f_{r+1,s-1}$ are marked by blue circles in the online version of Fig. 6.2. These double dependencies complicate the calculation of the f_{rs}: A specific sequence of calculations needs to be followed (see the answer to Question 6.o).

6.s The right-hand side of Eq. (6.90) is easily Laplace-transformed as we can just replace the ps by qs because terms like $A_{r+1}(s-1)$ can be treated as constants and can therefore be ignored in the integration needed for the Laplace transform. This yields, for the right-hand side of Eq. (6.90)

$$A_{r+1}(s-1)q_{r+1,s-1} + B(s+1)q_{r,s+1} - (A_r s + Bs)q_{rs}. \tag{6.148}$$

The only a little trickier part is the left-hand side—we have seen this, however, in the answer to Question 6.e. The only difference here is that we are faced with a *partial* derivative ($\frac{\partial p_{rs}}{\partial t}$), but we need $\frac{dp_{rs}}{dt}$ in order to obtain Whittle's result. As long as we assume that the other parameters of p are held constant (e.g. r, s, A_r, B, etc.), we can proceed as we did in the answer to Question 6.e using integration by parts. The only difference here is that for the first term of the integration by parts expression, the right-hand side of Eq. (6.130), $e^{-\lambda t} p_{rs}|_0^\infty$, we get $-\delta_{nr}\delta_{as}$. Here is the explanation:

- $e^{-\lambda t} p_{rs}$ vanishes as t approaches infinity, i.e. $t \to \infty$, resulting in 0.
- At $t = 0$ $p_{ns} = 1$, but $p_{rs} = 0$ for $r \neq n$ and $s \neq a$ resulting in the Kronecker Deltas, $\delta_{nr}\delta_{as}$ which are subtracted (the part of the evaluation of the definite integral which has to be subtracted).

Thus, we are left with

$$\int_{t=0}^{\infty} \frac{\partial p_{rs}}{\partial t} e^{-\lambda t} dt = \lambda q_{rs} - \delta_{nr}\delta_{as}. \tag{6.149}$$

Combining Eq. (6.149) with Eq. (6.148) we get

$$\lambda q_{rs} - \delta_{nr}\delta_{as} = A_{r+1}(s-1)q_{r+1,s-1} + B(s+1)q_{r,s+1} - (A_r s + Bs)q_{rs}. \tag{6.150}$$

Rearranging Eq. (6.150), in particular collecting the q_{rs} on the left-hand side and bringing $-\delta_{nr}\delta_{as}$ over to the right-hand side we get

$$(\lambda + A_r s + Bs)q_{rs} = A_{r+1}(s-1)q_{r+l,s-1} + B(s+1)q_{r,s+l} + \delta_{nr}\delta_{as},$$

which is the equation, (6.91), we were looking for.

6.t Let us multiply Eq. (6.102) by x^{s+1} and sum over s

$$\begin{aligned}
h_{rs}x^{s+1} &= \alpha_r h_{r,s+l}x^{s+1} + \beta_r h_{r+l,s-1}x^{s+1}, \\
\sum_{s=1}^{\infty} h_{rs}x^{s+1} &= \alpha_r \sum_{s=1}^{\infty} h_{r,s+l}x^{s+1} + \beta_r \sum_{s=1}^{\infty} h_{r+l,s-1}x^{s+1}, \\
H_r &= \frac{\alpha_r}{x} H_r - x\,\alpha_r h_{r,1} + \beta_r x\, H_{r+1} \text{ (see comments below)}, \\
H_r - \frac{\alpha_r}{x} H_r &= \beta_r x\, H_{r+1} - x\,\alpha_r h_{r1} \text{ (subtract } \frac{\alpha_r}{x} H_r \text{ from both sides)}, \\
H_r \left(\frac{x - \alpha_r}{x^2} \right) &= \beta_r H_{r+1} - \alpha_r h_{r1}, \\
H_r &= \frac{x^2}{x - \alpha_r} \left[\beta_r H_{r+1} - \alpha_r h_{r1} \right].
\end{aligned} \tag{6.151}$$

A few comments regarding the substitutions of the sums $\alpha_r \sum_{s=1}^{\infty} h_{r,s+l}x^{s+1}$ and $\beta_r \sum_{s=1}^{\infty} h_{r+l,s-1}x^{s+1}$ with the corresponding H:

1. $\sum_{s=1}^{\infty} h_{r,s+1}x^{s+1}$ is almost H_r, but not quite:

   a. We start summing from $s = 1$; therefore, we are missing the term $h_{r1}x^2$ because the sum is starting with h_{r2}. Thus, the term $h_{r1}x^2$ has to be subtracted to compensate for this deficit.

b. In the definition of H_r the exponent of x is one more than the subscript of the corresponding h_{rs}. That can be fixed by multiplying the sum by x.

Accordingly, the sum $\sum_{s=1}^{\infty} h_{r,s+1}x^{s+1}$ actually amounts to $\frac{H_r(x)-h_{r1}x^2}{x} = \frac{H_r(x)}{x} - h_{r1}x$.

6.u Eqs. (6.110), (6.111), and (6.112) give us the tools to recursively calculate the probabilities.

First, P_0, the probability that there are no secondary cases, has to be computed. For that we need $H_{n+1}(\alpha_n)$ which is given by Eq. (6.111):

$$H_{n+1}(\alpha_n) = \frac{\alpha_n^a}{A_{n+1}}.$$

Accordingly,

$$\begin{aligned}
P_0 &= B\frac{\beta_n}{\alpha_n}H_{n+1}(\alpha_n) && (6.152)\\
&= B\frac{\beta_n}{\alpha_n}\frac{\alpha_n^a}{A_{n+1}} && (6.153)\\
&= B\frac{\frac{A_{n+1}}{A_n+B}}{\frac{B}{A_n+B}}\frac{\left(\frac{B}{A_n+B}\right)^a}{A_{n+1}} && (6.154)\\
&= \left(\frac{B}{A_n+B}\right)^a. && (6.155)
\end{aligned}$$

We got from (6.154) to (6.155) by simplifying (canceling terms). Luckily, the term A_{n+1}—representing the transmission parameter given that there are $n+1$ susceptibles—in (6.153) disappears, and P_0 is easily calculated.

Just for the sake of the argument, let us assume that $B = 0.3$ (per day) and $A_r = 0.1\,r$ (per day—the constant 0.1 is multiplied by the number of susceptibles). Further I assume that $n = 10$ and that there is just one index case, i.e. $a = 1$. Plugging-in these values into Eq. (6.155), we get

$$P_0 = \left(\frac{0.3}{1+0.3}\right) = 0.231.$$

The probability that there will be no secondary transmission at all is 23%.

From here we can proceed as follows: Using P_0 we can calculate $H_{10}(\alpha_9)$ using (6.110) and (6.152); the latter is used to re-express $H_{11}(\alpha_{10})$ as

$$H_{11}(\alpha_{10}) = P_0\frac{\alpha_{10}}{\beta_{10}}\frac{1}{B} \tag{6.156}$$

and then, plugging that into Eq. (6.110),

$$\begin{aligned}
H_{10}(x) &= \frac{\beta_{10}x^2}{x-\alpha_{10}}\left[H_{11}(x) - H_{11}(\alpha_{10})\right]\\
&= \frac{\beta_{10}x^2}{x-\alpha_{10}}\left[\frac{x}{A_{n+1}} - P_0\frac{\alpha_{10}}{\beta_{10}}\frac{1}{B}\right]. && (6.157)
\end{aligned}$$

We simply substituted the expressions developed above for $H_{11}(x)$ (6.156) and $H_{11}(\alpha_{10})$ (6.111). To calculate P_1, the probability that there will be one single secondary case, we make use of Eq. (6.112) again, using the above expression for $H_{10}(x)$, (6.157), but substituting $\alpha_{n-w} = \alpha_9$ for x we get:

$$
\begin{aligned}
P_1 &= B\frac{\beta_9}{\alpha_9}H_{10}(\alpha_9) \\
&= B\frac{\beta_9}{\alpha_9}\frac{\beta_{10}\alpha_9^2}{\alpha_9-\alpha_{10}}\left[\frac{\alpha_9}{A_{11}} - P_0\frac{\alpha_{10}}{\beta_{10}}\frac{1}{B}\right] && (6.158) \\
&= B\frac{\frac{A_{10}}{A_9+B}}{\frac{B}{A_9+B}}\frac{\frac{A_{11}}{A_{10}+B}\left(\frac{B}{A_9+B}\right)^2}{\frac{B}{A_9+B}-\frac{B}{A_{10}+B}}\left[\frac{\frac{B}{A_9+B}}{A_{11}} - P_0\frac{\frac{B}{A_{10}+B}}{\frac{A_{11}}{A_{10}+B}}\frac{1}{B}\right] && (6.159) \\
&= \frac{A_{10}}{A_{10}-A_9}\frac{B}{A_9+B}\left[\frac{B}{A_9+B} - P_0\right]. && (6.160)
\end{aligned}
$$

Expression (6.160) is derived from (6.159) by simplifying and P_1 can now be calculated easily from the assumed values for B and A_9 and A_{10} and using the computed value for P_0. Thus we obtain $P_1 = 0.0475$.

6.v This is, admittedly, not a very profound question. As defined at the beginning of this section (page 136), A_r represents the transmission rate of one infectious individual in r susceptibles. For A_0, therefore, there are no susceptibles left, precluding the "production" of any new infected who can only be recruited among the susceptibles.

6.w Using Bailey's method, we have several choices of how to proceed. The simplest way is to go to his Table 2 ([2], p. 183) and look for the first entry under $n = 5$. The formula given is $P_0 = \rho/(\rho+5)$. But I didn't give you ρ in the question. Fortunately, that is easy to calculate using the definition of $\rho = B/A = 0.3/0.1 = 3$. Plugging this into the formula gives the result of $P_0 = 0.375$. Alternatively, we can use the double recursive algorithm, which is implemented in the online supplement, using R. The result, of course, will be the same.
To implement Whittle's method we utilize formula (6.155), $P_0 = B/(A_{n+1} + B)$ which gives the identical result.
Even though this was not asked for, we can compare computations for P_1 using Bailey's double recursive algorithm, or Eq. (6.160), using the corresponding values for n, $n-1$, and P_0.

Appendix 6.B Supplementary material

Supplementary material related to this chapter can be found online at http://dx.doi.org/10.1016/B978-0-12-802260-3.00006-7.

References

[1] N.T. Bailey, A simple stochastic epidemic, Biometrika (1950) 193–202.

[2] N.T. Bailey, The total size of a general stochastic epidemic, Biometrika 40 (1–2) (1953) 177–185.

[3] M. Bartlett, Some evolutionary stochastic processes, Journal of the Royal Statistical Society. Series B (Methodological) 11 (2) (1949) 211–229.

[4] D. Bernoulli, Essai d'une nouvelle analyse de la mortalité causée par lat petite Vérole, & des avantages de l'inoculation pour la prévenir, 1760.

[5] P. En'ko, On the course of epidemics of some infectious diseases, International Journal of Epidemiology 18 (4) (1989) 749–755.

[6] W.H. Hamer, The Milroy Lectures on Epidemic Disease in England: The Evidence of Variability and of Persistency of Type, Bedford Press, 1906.

[7] M. Kermack, A.G. McKendrick, Contributions to the mathematical theory of epidemics. Part I, Proceedings of the Royal Society. Series A, Containing Papers of a Mathematical and Physical Character 115 (5) (1927) 700–721.

[8] H. Soper, The interpretation of periodicity in disease prevalence, Journal of the Royal Statistical Society (1929) 34–73.

[9] P. Whittle, The outcome of a stochastic epidemic—a note on Bailey's paper, Biometrika 42 (1–2) (1955) 116–122.

[10] H.S. Wilf, generatingfunctionology, Elsevier, 2013.

O. Diekmann, J. Heesterbeek, and J.A. Metz (1991) and P. Van den Driessche and J. Watmough (2002): The spread of infectious diseases in heterogeneous populations

7

Contents

A Historical Introduction to Mathematical Modeling of Infectious Diseases. DOI: 10.1016/B978-0-12-802260-3.00007-9

7.1 Introduction: Non-homogeneous transmission

In this chapter we will take a big step, both in topic and time, by discussing two relatively recent papers. They both deal with transmission in heterogeneous population. All papers we have studied thus far assumed *homogeneous mixing*, i.e. that infectious contact in a population is unstructured: Each individual has the same probability of entering into (infectious) contact with anyone else.

Question 7.a

This kind of statement ("Each individual ...") would likely not raise many brows, although, depending on the context, at least two issues might be pointed out. Try to identify these issues when this statement is made in a "Kermack & McKendrick" context.

The point here is that, up to now, we made the simplifying assumption that everybody is, besides her/his infection status (susceptible, infected, etc.) exactly the same. This assumption was simply a convenient and reasonable simplification, and we never pretended that this was realistic. Now its time to move beyond that.

In this chapter, we will discuss two papers that discuss the treatment of transmission models for heterogeneous populations, with a focus on the basic reproduction number: The first paper is by Diekmann, Heesterbeek and Metz [1], a group from the Netherlands, and the second paper was written by van den Driesche and Watmough [6], Canada-based researchers. Both papers discuss the basic reproduction number, an enormously important epidemiologic quantity we have encountered before (Chap. 5), but here we take a more general approach to apply this to heterogeneous populations. We return to the world of ODE models and leave the stochastic and discrete world behind. Both papers are quite expansive, and we will consider only their first parts that introduce and derive the crucial elements.

7.2 Diekmann, Heesterbeek and Metz: The basic reproduction number in heterogeneous populations I

Diekmann and colleagues provide a brief introduction to their paper that is worth reading in its entirety. We just quote the most relevant passages here:

> *"Suppose we want to know whether or not a contagious disease can 'invade' into a population which is in a steady (at the time scale of disease transmission) demographic state with all individuals susceptible. To decide about this question we first of all* linearize, *i.e., we ignore the fact that the density of susceptibles decreases due to the infection process. It has become common practice in the analysis of the simplest models to consider next the associated* generation process *and to define the* basic reproduction ratio R_0 *as the* expected number of secondary cases *produced, in a completely susceptible population, by a* typical *infected individual during its entire period of infectiousness. The famous* threshold criterion *then states:*

the disease can invade if $R_0 > 1$, whereas it cannot if $R_0 < 1$.

It is the aim of this note to demonstrate how these ideas extend to less simple (though probably still highly oversimplified) models involving heterogeneity *in the population and to explain the meaning of 'typical' in the 'definition' of R_0 above."*

This is a nice introduction into what will follow. From here, the authors delve into the necessary definitions and begin by introducing a variable ξ, which is called h-state (h for heterogeneity) variable. What this means is this: ξ characterizes individuals' ability to infect others or to become infected by others. Specifically, infectivity is given by $A(\tau, \xi, \eta)$, the infectivity of an individual with h-state η that was infected τ time units ago for a susceptible individual with h-state ξ. Diekmann and colleagues refer to $A(\tau, \xi, \eta)$ as the "expected infectivity".

Question 7.b

Can you spot the notational "inconsistencies" in this paragraph that paraphrases Diekmann et al. (these inconsistencies are contained in the original text)?

The authors do not explicitly state what they mean by "infectivity". From what follows it becomes clear, however, that they are referring to the rate at which an infectious individual generates new infections *per* susceptible. They accomplish this by multiplying $A(\tau, \xi, \eta)$ with, say, $S(\xi)$, which represents the number of susceptibles with state ξ, the rate at which new infecteds of type ξ are generated by an infectious individual of type η, who has been infected for a duration of τ (probably in *days*, but we can choose whatever time units we like). Now, how many people will an infectious individual of h-type η produce in total? We have only seen the *rates*, $A(\tau, \xi, \eta)$, at which a certain infectious individual transmits the agent to susceptibles of certain type at a specific state of the "illness" (this is in quotes because we are not at this moment concerned whether there even *is* illness).

But to arrive at the required numbers, we have

1. To *integrate* the infectivity function over time, i.e. compute the "lifetime infectiousness" (this term is not used by Dieckmann et al.), given the "type" of the infectious and susceptible individual:

$$a_{\xi\eta} = \int_0^\infty A(\tau, \xi, \eta)\, d\tau. \tag{7.1}$$

   This is the *proportion of one* susceptible individual of h-type ξ infected by one infectious η individual during her/his infectious period. If you would call that quantity "odd", I might agree with you because fractions of individuals seem of little importance. However, we need to remind ourselves that we have left the realm of discrete stochastic models (Chap. 6) and are in the sphere of "continuous populations" that are devoid of individuals.
2. To quantify the total number of susceptible individuals of h-type ξ, there are $S(\xi)$ of them, that will be infected by one infectious η individual during her/his infectious period, we simply have to multiply $a_{\xi\eta}$ by $S(\xi)$ and get $S(\xi)\, a_{\xi\eta}$.

3. To *sum* (or integrate) over all types of susceptibles:

$$\int_{\Omega} S(\xi) \int_{0}^{\infty} A(\tau, \xi, \eta)\, d\tau d\xi. \tag{7.2}$$

The quantity is referred to by Diekmann et al. as *next generation factor*; I will use the term *next-generation factor* which is more commonly used in the literature.

7.2.1 A–more or less brief–detour

We now need to briefly discuss the use of integrals and sums. For the sake of generality, Diekmann et al. state, "[i]n order to have a unified notation for various cases we write integrals to denote sums whenever Ω is discrete (completely or just with respect to some component of ξ)" (*Remark*, p. 366). Ω, by the way, is the sample space of the h-states. Even though this breaks with my habit of following the original notation as closely as possible, I will use *sums* instead of integrals because that will make it easier for us to follow the exposition that follows. Diekmann et al. make use of linear operators, a generalization of matrices. This may be a good theoretical choice, but also perhaps an unnecessary complication. What follows now is therefore a deviation from Diekmann et al. that is intended to ease the understanding of their reasoning. We will later return to the original.

Here is the next-generation factor using a sum instead of the outer integral:

$$\sum_{\eta \in \Omega} S(\xi)\, a_{\eta\xi} = \sum_{\eta \in \Omega} S(\xi) \int_{0}^{\infty} A(\tau, \xi, \eta)\, d\tau. \tag{7.3}$$

Question 7.c

Interpret the "meaning" of the *next-generation factor*, i.e. explain that quantity.

Let us define the following vectors:

$$\mathbf{S} = \begin{bmatrix} S(1) \\ S(2) \\ \vdots \\ S(n) \end{bmatrix} \tag{7.4}$$

where the arguments of S, i.e. $1, 2, \ldots, n$, represent distinct h-types; so the vector $\mathbf{S}$ contains the numbers of susceptibles of any h-type. Similarly, we define

$$\mathbf{A}_{\eta} = \begin{bmatrix} a_{1\eta} \\ a_{2\eta} \\ \vdots \\ a_{n\eta} \end{bmatrix}. \tag{7.5}$$

Here, e.g. $a_{3\eta}$ represents the total amount of infectivity delivered by an infectious individual of h-type η, during his/her whole infectious period, to a susceptible individual of h-type 3. Using these two vectors, the next-generation factor can be written as

$$\mathbf{A}_\eta{}^T\,\mathbf{S}. \tag{7.6}$$

Following the rules of matrix multiplication, this corresponds to an element-wise multiplication and subsequent summation, exactly as in Eq. (7.3). To summarize the answer to Question 7.c (again), expression (7.6) captures the total number of infections caused by an infectious individual of type η.

Briefly returning to Diekmann et al., let us

> *"[...] abandon the idea of introducing an infected individual with a particular well-defined h-state and start instead with a 'distributed' individual described by a density ϕ." (p. 366, last paragraph)*

So, in order to have the transmission process captured in its complexity, we need a vector corresponding to (7.5) for *each* "infection-donating" h-type. Each of these vectors represents the portion of the *infectious* population as represented by the distribution $\phi(\eta)$.

Here, the term *distribution* represents a quasi statistical interpretation; a *statistical* interpretation would imply

$$\mathbf{\Phi} = \begin{bmatrix} \phi(1) \\ \phi(2) \\ \vdots \\ \phi(n) \end{bmatrix} \tag{7.7}$$

where $\phi(k) = \Pr(h\text{-type} = k)$ which reads: "The probability that the h-type of a, randomly selected, infectious individual, is k". Furthermore, $\|\mathbf{\Phi}\| = 1$, meaning the L_1-norm of the vector $\mathbf{\Phi}$, which simply is the sum of the absolute values of its elements, amounts to one. Note that the elements of $\mathbf{\Phi}$ *must* be non-negative because they represent *probabilities* and thus *must* equal their absolute value.

Here, however, we dwell in a deterministic world where probabilities have no place. A *quasi-statistical* meaning of *distribution* could be achieved by replacing *probability* with *proportion*: "The proportion of infectious individuals having h-type a". At the beginning of Section "1. The definition" (p. 366), Diekmann and colleagues state, for S that

> *"[...] in order to avoid confusion we emphasize that S is not a probability density function; that is, its integral equals the total population size in the steady demographic state, and not one."*

This alludes to a problem with the term "distribution" in this context, but in my opinion, the comment does really address the problem.

Let me here introduce the following $n \times n$ (square) matrix:

$$\mathbf{A_S} = \begin{bmatrix} a_{11}\,S(1) & a_{12}\,S(1) & \dots & a_{1n}\,S(1) \\ a_{21}\,S(2) & a_{22}\,S(2) & \dots & a_{2n}\,S(2) \\ \vdots & \vdots & \ddots & \vdots \\ a_{n1}\,S(n) & a_{n2}\,S(n) & \dots & a_{nn}\,S(n) \end{bmatrix}. \tag{7.8}$$

Let $\mathbf{A_S}[,\eta]$ denote the ηth column of $\mathbf{A_S}$ and $\mathbf{A_S}[\xi,]$ the ξth row of the matrix. The next-generation factor (7.6) could thus be expressed as the L_1-norm (the sum of the elements) of $\mathbf{A_S}[,\eta]$. I will call $\mathbf{A_S}$ the *next-generation matrix*.

Question 7.d

Show this, i.e. that the next-generation factor can be written as the L_1-norm of the ηth column of the matrix $\mathbf{A_S}$.

If we now want to compute the numbers of infectious individual of a specific h-type, say ξ, that are caused by our "distributed individual", we have to:

1. Compute, for each h-type ("infection-donor"), the numbers infections generated in susceptibles of specific h-type, e.g. ξ. To achieve this we multiply the numbers of susceptibles, here $S(\xi)$, with the respective lifetime infectiousness, say $a_{\xi\eta}$,
$$S(\xi)\,a_{\xi\eta}.$$
2. This number has to be weighted by the "number" of infectious individuals of h-type η; according to the scenario laid out by Diekmann and colleagues, we start out with only a proportion $\phi(\eta)$ of an individual being of type η,
$$S(\xi)\,a_{\xi\eta}\,\phi(\eta).$$
3. We have to sum over all h-types (infection donors), for example,
$$\sum_{\eta=1}^{n} S(\xi)\,a_{\xi\eta}\,\phi(\eta).$$

The step described in item **3.** can be accomplished using the ξth row of $\mathbf{A_S}$, namely $\mathbf{A_S}[\xi,]$,

$$\phi_1(\xi) = \sum_{\eta=1}^{n} S(\xi)\,a_{\xi\eta}\,\phi_0(\eta) = \mathbf{A_S}[\xi,]\,\mathbf{\Phi_0}. \tag{7.9}$$

The expression $\phi_1(\xi)$ is chosen to denote the *numbers* of new infections in individuals of h-type ξ originating from the "distributed" index case who is described by $\mathbf{\Phi_0}$. Ultimately, however, we would like to know how many new infections arise overall, in each of the h-types and, in particular, how that compares on average to the numbers in the preceding generation of infections. This can be accomplished by applying the approach implied by Eq. (7.9), but instead of using just *one* row of $\mathbf{A_S}$ using the full matrix:

$$\mathbf{\Phi_1} = \begin{bmatrix} \phi_1(1) \\ \phi_1(2) \\ \vdots \\ \phi_1(n) \end{bmatrix} = \mathbf{A_S}\,\mathbf{\Phi_0}. \tag{7.10}$$

As seen in the expression between the two '='-signs in (7.10), the elements of the resulting vector $\boldsymbol{\phi}_1$ represent calculations for specific h-states (susceptibles) as shown in Eq. (7.9). To reiterate, this vector represents the numbers of new infections, by h-state, resulting from the "distributed" individual.

Question 7.e

Consider the following expression:

$$\mathbf{\Phi_2} = \mathbf{A_S}\,\frac{\mathbf{\Phi_1}}{\|\mathbf{\Phi_1}\|}. \tag{7.11}$$

This would represent the equivalent to expression (7.10), but looking at the second generation of new infections, i.e. those originating from the "first generation" which, in turn originated from the "distributed" index case. Note that we divide $\mathbf{\Phi_1}$ by its norm to make it sum to one again. Is there anything that "bothers" you if you consider what would happen in a real outbreak? (Tip: This question has to do with $\mathbf{A_S}$.)

Let

$$\mathbf{\Phi_k} = \mathbf{A_S}\,\mathbf{\Phi_{k-1}}. \tag{7.12}$$

Then, interestingly, if we let n go to infinity, the following happens:

$$\lim_{k\to\infty} \mathbf{A_S}^k\,\mathbf{\Phi_0} = \varrho_d^k\, c\, \mathbf{\Phi_d}, \tag{7.13}$$

where ϱ_d and c are positive real numbers.

Question 7.f

First, translate the mathematical statement of (7.13) into English, i.e. interpret the meaning of that expression. Then, put it into context; use, e.g., expression (7.13) to connect it to related mathematical ideas.

In the answer to Question 7.f we saw that ϱ_d is the dominant eigenvalue of the matrix $\mathbf{A_S}$. How can we interpret this quantity in our context?

Putting it all together

As we have seen, if the distribution of the *index case(s)* is as given by $\mathbf{\Phi_d}$–or at least similar to it–then the next generation of infections will be distributed the same. Only, it will be augmented by a factor ϱ_d. In other words, each infectious individual will cause, averaged over all h states, ϱ_d secondary infections. If the population is *fully susceptible* as it is by definition (see discussion on *linearization* above), we arrive at the definition of R_0,

$$R_0 = \varrho_d. \tag{7.14}$$

7.2.2 Returning to the original

I will now return to where we left off the original text which, I believe, is easier to follow after the primer we just completed. However, we will revisit the derivation of R_0 using the "original" operator notations. The *next-generation operator* is given by

$$(K(S)\phi)(\xi) = S(\xi) \int_{\Omega} \int_{0}^{\infty} A(\tau, \xi, \eta) d\tau \phi(\eta) d\eta. \tag{7.15}$$

This equation quantifies the number of secondary cases of h-type ξ resulting from ϕ. Note that ϕ is a vector with the "amount" of all the h-types as entries ("distributed" individual).

> **Question 7.g**
>
> What expression, which we derived during our "detour", does the next-generation operator correspond (if the integral is replaced with a sum)?

Diekmann and colleagues continue that

> *"[...] we note that the next generation factor of ϕ is simply the $L_1(\Omega)$-norm of $K(S)\phi$, i.e.,*
>
> $$\int_{\Omega} S(\xi) \int_{\Omega} \int_{0}^{\infty} A(\tau, \xi, \eta) d\tau \phi(\eta) d\eta$$
>
> *[...] If we take the supremum of the next generation factor over all ϕ with $\|\phi\| = 1$ we obtain, by definition, the operator norm of $K(S)$." (p. 367)*

The $L_1(\Omega)$-norm of $K(S)\phi$ quantifies the number of cases resulting from an index case or index cases whose h-types (remember the "distributed individual") are represented by a particular ϕ. That particular configuration (= "distribution") of ϕ that yields the *most* secondary cases (= supremum), assuming that the susceptibles are not depleted,[1] represents the definition of the operator norm of $K(S)\phi$. The operator norm thus represents the upper limit of R_0: The average distribution may just be that ϕ that is associated with the supremum of $K(S)\phi$ which, in that case, would be the R_0. The R_0 could not be any higher.

A somewhat unfortunate example

As an example for the observation that the operator norm of $K(S)$ represents an *upper bound* of R_0, Diekmann et al. introduce a *host–vector model*. By vector, of course,

[1] See introduction of linearization on page 158.

they are referring to an *arthropod vector*, i.e. an arthropod[2] capable of transmitting an agent of disease, a topic Chap. 5 was devoted to. For this example, they choose $\Omega = \{1, 2\}$. Accordingly, there are *two* h-types, one corresponding to people, the other one to mosquitoes. The resulting linear operator or, as we called it, next-generation matrix is given by

$$K(S) = \begin{pmatrix} 0 & a_{12}\, S_1 \\ a_{21}\, S_2 & 0 \end{pmatrix}.$$

The operator norm $K(S)$ is given my $\max(a_{12}\, S_1, a_{21}\, S_2)$. This can be seen as follows. Assume two extreme cases: First, there is only h-type 1 (humans) such that the distribution is given by $\phi^T = (1, 0)$.[3] Calculation gives

$$K(S)\, \phi = \begin{pmatrix} 0 & a_{12}\, S_1 \\ a_{21}\, S_2 & 0 \end{pmatrix} \begin{bmatrix} 1 \\ 0 \end{bmatrix} = \begin{bmatrix} 0 \times 1 + 0 \times a_{12} \\ 1 \times a_{21} + 0 \times 0 \end{bmatrix} = \begin{bmatrix} 0 \\ a_{21} \end{bmatrix}. \tag{7.16}$$

The norm of $K(S)\, \phi$, which is a column vector, thus is $0 + a_{21} = a_{21}$; similarly, for the other case (only h-type 2, i.e. mosquitoes) the norm of $K(S)\, \phi$ will be $\|K(S)\, \phi\| = a_{12}$. The larger of the two will be the operator norm of $K(s)$. Diekmann and colleagues then write:

> *"These two numbers correspond to vector → host and host → vector transmission, respectively. No matter which of the two is the larger one, in the next generation it is necessarily the other of the two numbers which is the relevant* factor. *Therefore the operator norm of $K(S)$ is not a good definition of R_0. Since $a_{12}S_1a_{21}S_2$ is the two-generation factor, the average next generation factor is*
>
> $$\sqrt{a_{12}S_1a_{21}S_2}. \tag{7.17}$$
>
> *How can we define such a quantity in general?" (p. 367)*

Why a "somewhat unfortunate choice"?

The above example appears to serve its purpose. However, I disagree with this conception of vector-borne transmission. Heterogeneity clearly plays an important role in the transmission dynamics of many vector-borne agents. Constructing *arthropod vectors* (here mosquitoes) and *vertebrate hosts* (here people) as two different h-types, however, seems to me misguided as a_{ij} for $i = j$ is zero, i.e. such that transmission within h-type is not sustainable: Mosquitoes do not directly infect other mosquitoes and people do not directly infect other people. Well, mosquitoes can, in fact, in some cases infect other mosquitoes, *via* transovarial transmission of certain viruses, from infected female to offspring. We

[2] The phylum Arthropoda includes as diverse invertebrates as lobsters and butterflies–and, of course, mosquitoes and ticks.

[3] The vector representing the h-type distribution is a column vector. To conveniently write it as row vector, the vector has to be transposed, thus ϕ^T.

will return to this discussion when we will discuss this chapter's companion paper [6].

7.2.3 R_0–for the second time

In the previous section, Diekmann et al. asked how they could derive a generalized expression of (7.17), which was

$$\sqrt{a_{12}S_1a_{21}S_2},$$

and now continue to work out the answer:

> *"After m generations the magnitude of the infected population is (in the linear approximation) $K(S)^m\phi$ and consequently the per-generation growth factor is $\|K(S)^m\|^{1/m}$. We want to know what happens to the population in the long run, so we let $m \to \infty$." (p. 367)*

The answer to that question is actually equivalent (under the assumption that ϕ is discrete) to the result described by (7.13) where the linear operator was represented by a square matrix (Eq. (2.2) in [1]):

$$r(K(S)) = \inf_{m\geq 1} \|K(S)^m\|^{1/m} = \lim_{m\to\infty} \|K(S)^m\|^{1/m}. \tag{7.18}$$

Note that the *infimum* (inf) is, in many cases, equivalent with the *minimum*, the smallest value (e.g. smallest element of a closed set, such as $\{1, 2, 3, 4, 5\}$, the infimum of which would be 1).

$r(K(S))$ is called the spectral radius of $K(S)$. Importantly, $K(S)^m\phi$ converges to 0 if $r(K(S)) < 1$ and goes to infinity if $r(K(S)) > 1$. In fact, the spectral radius $r(K(S))$ is the *dominant eigenvalue* of $K(S)$, given certain technical conditions on A, S, and $K(\cdot)$. The *spectrum* of a square matrix is sometimes used to refer to all of the eigenvalues. The *spectral radius* is the eigenvalue with the *largest absolute value*. As we are dealing with *real* eigenvalues here, the *absolute eigenvalue* is just the eigenvalue itself.

Question 7.h

Could we have an intuition that the spectral radius, as defined in (7.18), is an *eigenvalue* of $K(S)$?

In analogy to (7.13), we can write

$$K(S)^m\phi \sim c(\phi)\varrho_d^m\phi_d \text{ for } m \to \infty \tag{7.19}$$

which could also be written as

$$\lim_{m\to\infty} K(S)^m\phi = c(\phi)\varrho_d^m\phi_d, \tag{7.20}$$

making the equivalence to expression (7.13) even more evident.

Diekmann et al. finish up this part of the paper by introducing the key definition of R_0:

Definition. $R_0 = r(K(S)) = \varrho_d =$ the dominant eigenvalue of $K(S)$ (p. 368),

where this is "the *typical* number of secondary cases."

7.2.4 From generations to time

The treatment of the epidemic process so far was based on a consideration of transmission generations. This approach is very intuitive for dealing with the basic reproduction number: If the population is fully susceptible, then the *index case(s)* (zeroth generation) must give rise to a first generation which is larger by the factor R_0 which, in turn, will give rise to the second generation, that is again increased by a factor R_0, etc. The problem is that transmission generations cannot be kept track of. What can be observed instead is the rate of appearance of new cases, i.e. the epidemic evolution. The authors comment on the above definition of the *basic reproduction number*:

> *"With this definition the threshold criterion remains valid, as can be verified as follows. The threshold criterion relates the generation process to the development of the epidemic in real time, both in the linearized version."*

presenting the following real-time expression for the infection rate

$$i(t,\xi) = S(\xi)\int_{\Omega}\int_0^{\infty} A(\tau,\xi,\eta)i(t-\tau,\eta)d\tau d\eta \text{ (Eq. (2.4) in the paper)} \qquad (7.21)$$

where $i(t,\xi)$ is the rate if infection in ξ-type individuals or, more precisely, individuals with h-type ξ, at time t. The right-hand side of (7.21), more specifically the inner integral, is a convolution integral (compare Chap. 4, Eq. (4.27)). The convolution integral captures the fact that the current rate of infection among ξ-type individuals depends on the number of *infecteds* of different h-types of different stage of infection which may bear upon their contagiousness. More specifically stated,

- New infections among individuals of h-type ξ are generated at a rate $i(t,\xi)$.
- Infections of h-class η that were generated τ time units ago have infectiousness $A(\tau,\xi,\eta)$ for subjects of type ξ.
- Thus these individuals contribute to the rate $i(t,\xi)$ the amount $A(\tau,\xi,\eta)i(t-\tau,\eta)$. Infections that may contribute to $i(t,\xi)$ were generated in the past, ranging from 0 to ∞ time units ago.
- In order to compile all these contributions, we have to integrate over the full time interval, i.e.

$$\int_0^{\infty} A(\tau,\xi,\eta)i(t-\tau,\eta)d\tau.$$

A linearized discrete version

If, on the other hand, infectiousness were an "on–off" phenomenon such that individuals are either infectious, possibly at levels depending on their h-type, or not and if we again assume discrete h-states, we could express the change in the numbers infected as

$$\frac{dI(t,\xi)}{dt} = a_{\xi,1}I(t,1) + a_{\xi,2}I(t,2) + \cdots + a_{\xi,n}I(t,n), \tag{7.22}$$

where $I(t,\eta)$ is the number of infectious subjects of h-type η at time t and $\eta \in \{1,\ldots,n\}$ ("η could be either 1 or 2, or ..., or n"); $a_{\xi,1},\ldots,a_{\xi,n}$ are transmission coefficients (real numbers) that also incorporate the numbers of susceptible. In the linearized situation, these numbers do not change (not in the paper).

Question 7.i

Obviously, Eqs. (7.21) and (7.22) look very different. Are they really different, though, in other ways than in their assumption regarding infectiousness over time ((7.21) allows for changing infectiousness while (7.22) assumes constant infectiousness) and the discrete h-states in (7.22)? Is there anything funny about this equation that appears strange to you, especially if you recall the chapter on Kermack & McKendrick's famous paper?

Solution to the real-time equation

The authors remark on Eq. (7.21) that it

> *"[...] has a solution of the form $i(t,\xi) = e^{\lambda t}\psi(\xi)$ if and only if ψ is an eigenvector of the operator K_λ*
>
> $$(K_\lambda\phi)(\xi) = S(\xi)\int_\Omega\int_0^\infty A(\tau,\xi,\eta)\,e^{-\lambda\tau}d\tau\,\phi(\eta)\,d\eta \tag{7.23}$$
>
> *with eigenvalue one." (p. 368)*

These statements warrant some comments:

1. The fact that this system of equations—there is one equation for each h-state—may have a solution of the form

$$i(t,\xi) = e^{\lambda t}\psi(\xi) \tag{7.24}$$

is explained by its linearization. *Linear* systems of differential equations do not have nonlinear terms, such as products of two variables. Exactly such products are key elements of equations as the ones brought to fame by Kermack & McKendrick. Consider the following linear system:

$$\dot{\mathbf{x}} = \mathbf{A}\mathbf{x},$$

where $\mathbf{x}$ is the k-sized vector of variables, e.g. $x_1, x_2, \ldots, x_k$, and $\mathbf{A}$ is the $k \times k$ coefficient matrix; $\dot{\mathbf{x}}$ refers to the derivatives with respect to time. This system has a solution of the form

$$\mathbf{x} = e^{\lambda t}\mathbf{v},$$

where λ is an eigenvalue of $\mathbf{A}$ and $\mathbf{v}$ is the corresponding eigenvector. If infectiousness is constant over time, such that the change in infectious individuals is determined by the *numbers* of infectious individuals of various h-types, such a solution could be found.

2. Two references [3,4] are given for the mentioned conditions for the solution, based on the operator (7.23), one for the general case and one for the discrete case. I do not find these texts particularly revealing and leave it at my assessment that this is another example of the obscure writing that ultimately motivated this book.

Where did operator K_λ come from?

This is not quite obvious and no assistance is offered by Diekmann and colleagues. However, consider the equation for i, (7.21); let us use the general solution for i (7.24) in that equation:

$$\begin{aligned}
i(t,\xi) &= S(\xi)\int_\Omega\int_0^\infty A(\tau,\xi,\eta)\, i(t-\tau,\eta)\, d\tau\, d\eta, \\
e^{\lambda t}\psi(\xi) &= S(\xi)\int_\Omega\int_0^\infty A(\tau,\xi,\eta)\, e^{\lambda(t-\tau)}\, \psi(\eta)\, d\tau\, d\eta \qquad (7.25)\\
&= S(\xi)\int_\Omega\int_0^\infty A(\tau,\xi,\eta)\, e^{\lambda t}\, e^{-\lambda\tau}\psi(\eta)\, d\tau\, d\eta\ (e^{\lambda(t-\tau)} = e^{\lambda t}\, e^{-\lambda\tau}),\\
\psi(\xi) &= S(\xi)\int_\Omega\int_0^\infty A(\tau,\xi,\eta)\, e^{-\lambda\tau}\, \psi(\eta)\, d\tau\, d\eta\ (\text{divide by } e^{\lambda t})\\
&= S(\xi)\int_\Omega\int_0^\infty A(\tau,\xi,\eta)\, e^{-\lambda\tau}\, d\tau\, \psi(\eta)\, d\eta. \qquad (7.26)
\end{aligned}$$

To get the last equation (7.26), we took $\psi(\eta)$ outside the inner integral because it does not involve time τ. So what expression (7.26) captures is how the distribution of infectious of h-type ξ changes as a function of infections in all the other h-types. The right-hand side is the operator we were looking for.

If ψ is an eigenvector of that operator, the operator multiplies that vector by a number (= eigenvalue). Intuitively, we can see that any *growth* (or decline) that would be brought on ψ by the operator is counteracted by the factor $e^{\lambda\tau}$, effectively forcing the eigenvalue to be one.

(Concluding) remarks

The authors continue that "Positivity arguments can be used to show that among the set of such λ with largest real part there is a real one, which we shall denote by λ_d (and the corresponding eigenvector by ψ_d). Monotonicity arguments then imply that

$$\lambda_d > 0 \Leftrightarrow R_0 > l \text{ and } \lambda_d < 0 \Leftrightarrow R_0 < l. \qquad (7.27)$$

The authors conclude Sect. 2 of the article ("The definition") by seven *Remarks* (bottom of p. 368). Not all of these remarks are equally relevant, and I will comment only on a few:

1. "Whereas R_0 is a number, λ_d is a rate." This statement refers to the threshold criteria (7.27). In fact, the basic reproduction number, occasionally referred to as "basic reproductive *rate*" or similarly, is *not* a rate and has no units. The parameter λ, on the other hand, represents an "epidemic growth rate" ($\lambda > 0$) or "epidemic decay rate" ($\lambda < 0$), respectively; see Eq. (7.24).

2. λ_d and ψ_d describe the exponential phase of an epidemic. If they are used in Eq. (7.24):

$$i(t, \xi) = e^{\lambda_d t} \psi_d(\xi), \tag{7.28}$$

the exponential term represents exponential growth (or decay). The vector ψ_d, on the other hand, captures the "average" h-state distribution. Diekmann et al. refer to that when they say that the "precise manner in which the epidemic started has died off."

5. If a model includes death and birth rates and both are—if affected at all—*negatively* affected (death rate *up*, birth rate *down*) then "[...] one can prove, in general, *global* rather than local stability for $R_0 < 1$. Or, in other words, endemic states are impossible when $R_0 > 1$." This is actually disputed even in the title of our next paper [6] ("...sub-threshold endemic equilibria ..."), but we will touch on that only briefly at the end of the next section because of fundamental doubts regarding the process by which that insight had been received.

6. If the system is in an endemic state, such that the number of susceptibles is $\hat{S}$, then $r(K(\hat{S})) = 1$, "necessarily". Clearly, in the endemic state, the epidemic does not grow.

We have only made it through the first 4 or 5 pages of this paper, which is barely a third, although the most important part. The paper continues with special cases and examples. Most of the material should be accessible to the reader with the background acquired thus far, and I recommend to the reader at least to browse through the remainder of the paper. We continue instead with the discussion of the second paper.

7.3 P. Van den Driessche and J. Watmough: Reproduction numbers and sub-threshold endemic equilibria for compartmental models of disease transmission

This paper by P. Van den Driessche and J. Watmough, like the paper by Diekmann and colleagues, focuses on the formulation of the basic reproduction number, but develops a more general framework for the study of the stability of transmission systems. While Diekmann et al. drew heavily on operator theory, van den Driessche and Watmough make use of dynamic systems theory, yet another branch of mathematics.

7.3.1 The model

The model which is developed here is more general than the models we have seen elsewhere. The population is divided up into n compartments that are differentiated by arbitrary characteristics, but the compartments are homogeneous, basically meaning that, in a given compartment, "everybody is the same".

Question 7.j

I purposely did not describe any characteristics because pondering the kind of characteristics they may be referring to is a useful exercise.

Van den Driessche and Watmough then formulate the following definitions and assumptions:

1. Let $x = (x_1, \ldots, x_n)^T$, for $x_i \geq 0$. Two comments:
   - **a.** x is a column vector; the transposition of that vector, denoted by "$()^T$", simply allows the vector to be displayed on a line.
   - **b.** The condition that x_i has to be non-negative follows from the model which represents *individuals.*
2. The n compartments are ordered, such that the first m compartments represent *infected* compartments.
3. $\mathbf{X}_s$ denotes the set of *all disease free states*, i.e.

$$\mathbf{X}_s = \{x \geq 0 | x_i = 0, i = 1, \ldots, m\}. \tag{7.29}$$

4. Let $\mathscr{F}_i$ be the rate of appearance of *new infections* in compartment i, for $i = 1, \ldots, m$, as only compartments up to m harbor infected individuals;
5. $\mathscr{V}_i = \mathscr{V}_i^- - \mathscr{V}_i^+$, where $\mathscr{V}_i^-$ is the transfer out of compartment i and $\mathscr{V}_i^+$ is the transfer into that compartment by any other means.

The model is then formulated as

$$\dot{x}_i = f_i(x) = \mathscr{F}_i(x) - \mathscr{V}_i(x), \qquad i = 1, \ldots, n. \tag{7.30}$$

The notation $\dot{x}$ refers to the derivative with respect to time, i.e.

$$\dot{x} = \frac{dx}{dt}. \tag{7.31}$$

An exemplary model

It will help us understand some of the concepts and derivations if we can *look* at a model. Further along in this paper, the authors actually provide several examples of heterogeneous models, but I prefer to set up a model that is as simple as possible while still offering generalization to the classical Kermack & McKendrick model to aid the illustration of the exposition that follows:

$$\dot{x}_1 = -\beta_{11}x_1y_1 - \beta_{21}x_1y_2, \tag{7.32}$$
$$\dot{x}_2 = -\beta_{12}x_2y_1 - \beta_{22}x_2y_2, \tag{7.33}$$
$$\dot{y}_1 = \beta_{11}x_1y_1 + \beta_{21}x_1y_2 - \gamma_1y_1, \tag{7.34}$$
$$\dot{y}_2 = \beta_{21}x_2y_1 + \beta_{22}x_2y_2 - \gamma_2y_2, \tag{7.35}$$

where x_1, x_2 are two types of susceptibles that, upon infection, turn into two types of infectious, y_1, y_2. Transmission is driven by type-specific transmission parameters,

β_{jk} (from infected of type j to susceptible k). Infectious types are removed at a rate governed by, again possibly type-specific, removal parameters γ_j. We assume that $N_1 = x_1 + y_1$ and $N_2 = x_2 + y_2$ are constant. We therefore do not have to write down the equations for the *removed* compartments as they are redundant: $r_1 = N_1 - x_1 - y_1$ and similarly for r_2. To make this model compatible with the notation of the paper, I relabel the infectious:

$$\dot{x}_1 = \beta_{11}x_1x_3 + \beta_{21}x_2x_3 - \gamma_1 x_1, \tag{7.36}$$

$$\dot{x}_2 = \beta_{12}x_1x_4 + \beta_{22}x_2x_4 - \gamma_2 x_2, \tag{7.37}$$

$$\dot{x}_3 = -\beta_{11}x_1x_3 - \beta_{21}x_2x_3, \tag{7.38}$$

$$\dot{x}_4 = -\beta_{12}x_1x_4 - \beta_{22}x_2x_4. \tag{7.39}$$

Note that x_1, x_2 turned into x_3, x_4 and y_1, y_2 have become x_1, x_2. To facilitate the discussion, especially of Assumption (A5), I introduce the following more general notation of the system (7.36)–(7.39) that makes use of the functions $\mathscr{F}$ and $\mathscr{V}$:

$$\dot{x}_1 = \mathscr{F}_1(x) - \mathscr{V}_1(x), \tag{7.40}$$

$$\dot{x}_2 = \mathscr{F}_2(x) - \mathscr{V}_2(x), \tag{7.41}$$

$$\dot{x}_3 = -\mathscr{V}_3(x), \tag{7.42}$$

$$\dot{x}_4 = -\mathscr{V}_4(x). \tag{7.43}$$

The function $\mathscr{F}$ does not appear in Eqs. (7.42) and (7.43) because of Assumption (A3) (see below). What these functions exactly are is left as a question (Question 7.k, below). An even more compact way of writing this system is the following:

$$\dot{x} = f(x). \tag{7.44}$$

In Eq. (7.44), x is the vector $x = (x_1, \ldots, x_4)^T$ which represents numbers in compartments 1 through 4. The left-hand side of (7.44), $\dot{x}$, represents the derivatives of x with respect to time.

The function $f(x) = \mathscr{F}(x) - \mathscr{V}(x)$ takes inputs from all compartments and outputs a vector of the same size, specifically the derivatives $\dot{x}_1$, $\dot{x}_2$, $\dot{x}_3$, and $\dot{x}_4$.

Five assumptions

Van den Driessche and Watmough formulate five assumptions regarding the functions $\mathscr{F}, \mathscr{V}^-$, and $\mathscr{V}^+$. I will first simply state these assumptions–mostly closely paraphrased–and will then comment and explain:

(A1) If $x \geq 0$, then $\mathscr{F}_i^-, \mathscr{V}_i^+, \mathscr{V}_i^- \geq 0$ for $i = 1, \ldots, n$. The functions $\mathscr{F}$ and $\mathscr{V}$ must be non-negative because, as the authors write, they represent a "directed transfer of individuals" (p. 31).

Question 7.k

Write down the functions $\mathscr{F}$ and $\mathscr{V}$ for our model (Eqs. (7.32)–(7.35)).

Due to the continuous nature of this model, the interpretation of x as "individuals" can be disputed, as I have done elsewhere, but this is not the point here.

(A2) If $x_i = 0$ then $\mathscr{V}_i^- = 0$. In particular, if $x \in \mathbf{X_s}$ the $\mathscr{V}_i^- = 0$ for $i = 1, \ldots, m$. This simply says that nothing can be transferred out of an empty compartment.

(A3) $\mathscr{F}_i = 0$ for $i > m$. This assumption only states that "uninfected compartments" remain uninfected. This has to do with the structure of the model: Clearly, if we define compartment as *susceptible*, for example, it cannot accommodate new infections. Therefore, the function $\mathscr{F}$ will give zero for uninfected compartments, and the corresponding terms will be dropped from Eqs. (7.42) and (7.43).

(A4) If $x \in \mathbf{X_s}$ then $\mathscr{F}_i(x) = 0$ and $\mathscr{V}_i^+ = 0$ for $i = 1, \ldots, m$. This assumption states that a disease-free population will stay disease-free.

(A5) If $\mathscr{F}(x)$ is set to zero, then all eigenvalues of $Df(x_0)$ have negative real parts. This assumption merits its own section.

Assumption 5: Linearization and the Jacobian

The last assumption, (A5), is focused on derivatives of f near the *disease-free equilibrium* (DFE). The authors briefly discuss the important DFE concept in the introduction section: The DFE is the state of the model where the population remains disease-free. This is clearly the case when the compartments representing infected individuals are empty.

We have encountered *linearized systems* before, specifically earlier in this chapter, but also elsewhere. Intuitively, linearization of a nonlinear system is achieved by setting certain dynamic quantities constant: On page 158 of this chapter we linearized by leaving the number of susceptibles constant; this may be a reasonable simplifying assumption if there are *many* susceptibles and their decline initially is barely noticeable.

More mathematically speaking, a *linearized* nonlinear system represents a *linear approximation*, which, in the one-dimensional case (only *one* variable), can be written as

$$f(x) \approx f(a) + f'(a)(x - a). \tag{7.45}$$

This is an approximation to the function $f(x)$ in the neighborhood of a (i.e. close to a), assuming that we know the value of the function at a, as well as the value of the first derivative of the function evaluated at a. Eq. (7.45) is derived from a *first-order Taylor polynomial*. In the following question, an example is given.

Question 7.I

Compute the linear approximation of

$$f(x) = x^2$$

in the neighborhood of 3: for $x = 3.1$, $x = 3.2$, and $x = 4$ and comment on your results.

The equivalent procedure for a multi-dimensional (*many*, e.g. k, variables) vector-valued (returns a $k \times 1$ vector) function is given by

$$\dot{x} = Df(x_0)(x - x_0), \tag{7.46}$$

where

$$Df(x_0) = \begin{bmatrix} \partial f_1/\partial x_1 & \partial f_1/\partial x_2 & \dots & \partial f_1/\partial x_n \\ \partial f_2/\partial x_1 & \partial f_2/\partial x_2 & \dots & \partial f_2/\partial x_n \\ \vdots & \vdots & \ddots & \vdots \\ \partial f_n/\partial x_1 & \partial f_n/\partial x_2 & \dots & \partial f_n/\partial x_n \end{bmatrix} \tag{7.47}$$

is the *Jacobian matrix* of $f(x)$, evaluated at x_0. In the matrix in Eq. (7.47) I omitted the "evaluated at x_0" argument from the partial derivatives for simplicity. Note that this linearized system in the neighborhood of the *fixed point,* or equilibrium point, where $\dot{x} = 0$ describes the behavior under perturbation, i.e. when the system is brought out of equilibrium, i.e. away from x_0.

A Jacobian matrix is the matrix of all partial derivatives (first order) of a vector-valued function. Just to make the analogy to (7.45) more obvious, Eq. (7.46) can be written in the following form:

$$f(x) \approx f(x_0) + Df(x_0)(x - x_0), \tag{7.48}$$

where $f(x) = \dot{x}$ (Eq. (7.44)). As x_0 represents the DFE,

$$f(x_0) = 0$$

as the "disease-free equilibrium" implies "nothing changes" and $f(x) = \dot{x}$ describes the rate of change in x over time. Therefore, the linearized system becomes (7.46), i.e.

$$\dot{x} = Df(x_0)(x - x_0).$$

As the authors point out, the attention is restricted to systems that are stable in the absence of new infections. To better understand this statement, as well as (A5), we have to take another detour, to think about model stability and eigenvalues.

Model stability and eigenvalues of the Jacobian matrix

How is the negativity of eigenvalues of the *Jacobian matrix*, in particular of their *real parts* (see the next section), related to a systems stability? Why are we only looking at systems "that are stable in the absence of new infections" and how is that related to (A5)?

To someone not intimately familiar with dynamical systems theory these statements may appear exceedingly obscure. Such statements, however, are well common territory in dynamical systems theory and stability analysis. I do not offer a formal proof, but show an intuitive explanation:

Consider the following simple linear system:

$$\begin{aligned} \dot{x}_1 &= a_1x_1 + b_1x_2 + c_1x_3 + d_1x_4, \\ \dot{x}_2 &= a_2x_1 + b_2x_2 + c_2x_3 + d_2x_4, \\ \dot{x}_3 &= a_3x_1 + b_3x_2 + c_3x_3 + d_3x_4, \\ \dot{x}_4 &= a_4x_1 + b_4x_2 + c_4x_3 + d_4x_4. \end{aligned}$$

If we define $x = [x_1, x_2, x_2, x_4]^T$, x is the column vector consisting of the four x_is as we have seen in our model. Let the coefficient matrix be

$$A = \begin{bmatrix} a_1 & b_1 & c_1 & d_1 \\ a_2 & b_2 & c_2 & d_2 \\ a_3 & b_3 & c_3 & d_3 \\ a_4 & b_4 & c_4 & d_4 \end{bmatrix}. \tag{7.49}$$

Using rules of linear algebra, we can write this simple system as

$$\dot{x} = Ax. \tag{7.50}$$

As can be seen in any textbook on differential equations, the general solution to this linear system is of the following form:

$$x = \alpha_1 v_1 e^{\lambda_1 t} + \alpha_2 v_2 e^{\lambda_2 t} + \alpha_3 v_3 e^{\lambda_3 t} + \alpha_4 v_4 e^{\lambda_4 t}, \tag{7.51}$$

where $\alpha_1, \ldots, \alpha_4$ are constants, $\lambda_1, \ldots, \lambda_4$ are the four eigenvalues of A and $v_1, \ldots, v_4$ the associated eigenvectors. Any of the $ve^{\lambda t}$ are also solutions to the system. If any of the four eigenvalues are positive, for that particular solution, x will increase with increasing time t and ultimately go to infinity. If, on the other hand, all of the eigenvalues are *negative*, x will always tend to zero with increasing t.

To understand why that corresponds to what we wanted to show, we have to remind ourselves of the context: In our case, we linearized the nonlinear system $\dot{x} = f(x)$ in the neighborhood of an equilibrium or *fixed point* to $\dot{x} = Df(x_0)(x - x_0)$. We define the following change of variable:

$$x^* = x - x_0. \tag{7.52}$$

This allows us to write (7.46) as

$$\dot{x} = Df(x_0)\, x^*. \tag{7.53}$$

Question 7.m

To get Eq. (7.53) from (7.46), we obviously just swapped $(x - x_0)$ for x^*, using the change of variable (7.52) on the right-hand side. Why is (7.53) analogous to the simple model (7.50), even though we have $\dot{x}$ instead of $\dot{x}^*$ on the left-hand side?

As we have shown, in the answer to Question 7.m, that (7.51) can be used with (7.46) if we rewrite that equation as

$$\dot{x}^* = Df(x_0)\, x^*,$$

we can use the above result as follows: If the Jacobian $Df(x_0)$ of the linearized system

$$\dot{x} = Df(x_0)\,(x - x_0),$$

evaluated at the fixed point x_0, has only negative real eigenvalues, then, in the neighborhood of x_0, the system is stable. This is because if the system is, at least "slightly" perturbed to x^*, such that it is at x, x^* will tend to zero, which is to say x will tend to x_0, the fixed point and the system will return to the fixed point.

Doing the calculations—first try

To get to grips with this, let us calculate the Jacobian, evaluated at x_0, for our simple model (7.50). To obtain that, we have to compute the *partial derivatives* of $f_1, \ldots, f_4$ at x_0, which are the left-hand side expressions of (7.50), with respect to all the variables, $x_1, \ldots, x_4$. Let me demonstrate this only for two elements of the matrix (7.47):

1. Using the right-hand side of the first equation of (7.50) with the basic rules of derivatives, the first element of the first row of (7.47) is

$$\begin{aligned}\frac{\partial f_1}{\partial x_1} &= \frac{\partial(\beta_{11}x_1x_3 + \beta_{21}x_2x_3 - x_1\gamma_1)}{\partial x_1} \\ &= \beta_{11}x_3 - \gamma_1. \end{aligned} \tag{7.54}$$

2. Similarly, the second element of the second row of (7.47) is

$$\begin{aligned}\frac{\partial f_2}{\partial x_2} &= \frac{\partial(\beta_{12}x_1x_4 + \beta_{22}x_2x_4 - x_2\gamma_2)}{\partial x_2} \\ &= \beta_{22}x_4 - \gamma_2. \end{aligned} \tag{7.55}$$

Continuing in a similar fashion with the other elements, we get

$$Df(x) = \begin{bmatrix} \beta_{11}x_3 - \gamma_1 & \beta_{21}x_3 & \beta_{11}x_1 + \beta_{21}x_2 & 0 \\ \beta_{12}x_4 & \beta_{22}x_4 - \gamma_2 & 0 & \beta_{12}x1 + \beta_{22}x_2 \\ -\beta_{11}x_3 & -\beta_{21}x_3 & -\beta_{11}x_1 - \beta_{21}x_2 & 0 \\ -\beta_{12}x_4 & -\beta_{22}x_4 & 0 & -\beta_{12}x_1 - \beta_{22}x_2 \end{bmatrix}. \tag{7.56}$$

However, as we need $Df(x_0)$, the Jacobian evaluated at x_0, which in our case is the DFE, i.e. with all infected compartments empty ($x_1 = x_2 = 0$), (7.56) becomes, setting all terms involving x_1, x_2 to zero,

$$Df(x_0) = \begin{bmatrix} \beta_{11}x_3 - \gamma_1 & \beta_{21}x_3 & 0 & 0 \\ \beta_{12}x_4 & \beta_{22}x_4 - \gamma_2 & 0 & 0 \\ -\beta_{11}x_3 & -\beta_{21}x_3 & 0 & 0 \\ -\beta_{12}x_4 & -\beta_{22}x_4 & 0 & 0 \end{bmatrix}. \tag{7.57}$$

Now we can proceed to calculate the eigenvalues of the matrix (7.57). How to calculate eigenvalues is outlined in any linear algebra textbook. What may seem very obscure can easily be understood from basic principles. We leave it to the reader to revisit that topic.

Basically, to compute the four eigenvalues of the 4×4 matrix

$$A = \begin{bmatrix} a_1 & b_1 & c_1 & d_1 \\ a_2 & b_2 & c_2 & d_2 \\ a_3 & b_3 & c_3 & d_3 \\ a_4 & b_4 & c_4 & d_4 \end{bmatrix}, \tag{7.58}$$

we subtract the matrix

$$\lambda I = \begin{bmatrix} \lambda & 0 & 0 & 0 \\ 0 & \lambda & 0 & 0 \\ 0 & 0 & \lambda & 0 \\ 0 & 0 & 0 & \lambda \end{bmatrix} \tag{7.59}$$

from A to give

$$A - \lambda I = \begin{bmatrix} a_1 - \lambda & b_1 & c_1 & d_1 \\ a_2 & b_2 - \lambda & c_2 & d_2 \\ a_3 & b_3 & c_3 - \lambda & d_3 \\ a_4 & b_4 & c_4 & d_4 - \lambda \end{bmatrix}. \tag{7.60}$$

Setting the determinant of $A - \lambda I$ to zero (characteristic equation), we can solve for λ. For readers rusty in linear algebra, I recommend to briefly read about that important topic.

Returning to our example, the characteristic equation is

$$\begin{vmatrix} \beta_{11}x_3 - \gamma_1 - \lambda & \beta_{21}x_3 & 0 & 0 \\ \beta_{12}x_4 & \beta_{22}x_4 - \gamma_2 - \lambda & 0 & 0 \\ -\beta_{11}x_3 & -\beta_{21}x_3 & -\lambda & 0 \\ -\beta_{12}x_4 & -\beta_{22}x_4 & 0 & -\lambda \end{vmatrix} = \mathbf{0}. \tag{7.61}$$

The **0** on the right-hand side of (7.61) is a vector of zeros. The vertical bars on the left-hand side are the common notation for a matrix determinant. So we can compute eigenvalues, I assume values for the βs and the xs:

$$\begin{aligned} \beta_{11} &= 0.001, \\ \beta_{12} &= 0.0005, \\ \beta_{21} &= 0.0005, \\ \beta_{22} &= 0.001, \\ x_3 &= 100, \\ x_4 &= 100. \end{aligned}$$

Plugging in these values into the characteristic equation (7.61), we get the following equation:

$$\begin{vmatrix} -0.40 - \lambda & 0.5 & 0 & 0 \\ 0.5 & -0.40 - \lambda & 0 & 0 \\ -0.10 & -0.05 & 0 - \lambda & 0 \\ -0.05 & -0.10 & 0 & 0 - \lambda \end{vmatrix} = \mathbf{0}. \tag{7.62}$$

There are online resources that calculate characteristic polynomials, eigenvalues, and eigenvectors (e.g. http://www.mathportal.org/calculators/matrices-calculators/matrix-calculator.php). I used the named resource to calculate the characteristic polynomial, but I also checked it by hand. The resulting characteristic polynomial is

$$p(x) = \lambda^4 + 0.6\lambda^3 + 0.63\lambda^2. \tag{7.63}$$

The corresponding eigenvalues are:

$$\lambda_1 = -0.45, \quad (7.64)$$
$$\lambda_2 = -0.35, \quad (7.65)$$
$$\lambda_3 = 0, \quad (7.66)$$
$$\lambda_4 = 0. \quad (7.67)$$

This result is in clear contradiction to (A5), which postulates that "If $\mathscr{F}(x)$ is set to zero, then all eigenvalues of $Df(x_0)$ have negative real parts." We did set $\mathscr{F}(x)$ to zero, simply by setting the infectious compartments to zero, which corresponds to our DFE. Clearly, if there are no infectious "individuals", no new infections can arise, thus $\mathscr{F}(x) = 0$. Nevertheless, not all of the eigenvalues of the Jacobian of our system, evaluated at x_0 (= DFE), are negative; two eigenvalues are zero. This complicates the situation, as local stability can no longer be evaluated using the sign of the real parts of the eigenvalues. Briefly, our model does not meet Assumption (A5).

Question 7.n

Do you have an idea what might be "wrong" here, i.e. why our simple model does not meet (A5)? Hint: Look at the Jacobian and try figuring out why columns 3 and 4 are zero.

Let us therefore modify our model so it meets all assumptions.

A second model and doing the calculations—second try

A modified, "proper" model which is compatible with assumption could be the following:

$$\dot{x}_1 = \beta_{11}x_1x_3 + \beta_{21}x_2x_3 - (\gamma_1 + \mu_1)x_1, \quad (7.68)$$
$$\dot{x}_2 = \beta_{12}x_1x_4 + \beta_{22}x_2x_4 - (\gamma_2 + \mu_2)x_2, \quad (7.69)$$
$$\dot{x}_3 = -\beta_{11}x_1x_3 - \beta_{21}x_2x_3 + (\rho_1 - \mu_1)x_3 + (N_1 - x_3)\rho_1, \quad (7.70)$$
$$\dot{x}_4 = -\beta_{12}x_1x_4 - \beta_{22}x_2x_4 + (\rho_2 - \mu_2)x_4 + (N_2 - x_4)\rho_2. \quad (7.71)$$

Now, we also assume *mortality* which may be different for the different type of people, but not affected by infection (μ_1, μ_2) as well as a "renewal" process, for example, by births that replenish the susceptibles. As we do not keep track of the recovered immune class, I also have to introduce the total number of susceptibles of either type, N_1, N_2. The two expressions $(N_1 - x_3)$ and $(N_2 - x_4)$ capture the infectious and removed.[4] For the following calculations, let me assign the following values to the new parameters: $\mu_1 = 0.001$, $\mu_2 = 0.001$, $\rho_1 = 0.001$, and $\rho_2 = 0.001$ (see online supplement for numerical solution to these two models).

[4] N_1 is composed of all susceptibles, infecteds, and removed of type 1, and the equivalent is true for N_2.

The Jacobian evaluated at the DFE, i.e. with $x_1 = x_2 = 0$, is

$$Df(x_0) = \begin{bmatrix} \beta_{11}x_3 - (\gamma_1 + \mu_1) & \beta_{21}x_3 & 0 & 0 \\ \beta_{12}x_4 & \beta_{22}x_4 - (\gamma_2 - \mu_2) & 0 & 0 \\ -\beta_{11}x_3 - \rho_1 & -\beta_{21}x_3 & -\mu_1 & 0 \\ -\beta_{12}x_4 & -\beta_{22}x_4 - \rho_2 & 0 & -\mu_2 \end{bmatrix}. \tag{7.72}$$

Also using the parameter and variable values from before gives

$$Df(x_0) = \begin{bmatrix} -0.401 & 0.050 & 0 & 0 \\ 0.050 & -0.401 & 0 & 0 \\ -0.101 & -0.050 & -0.001 & 0 \\ -0.050 & -0.101 & 0 & -0.001 \end{bmatrix}. \tag{7.73}$$

The eigenvalues are calculated using the *eigen* function in R (see online Supplement—also for the numerical solutions to the two models): −0.45, −0.35, −0.001, and −0.001 which are all real and negative and thus fulfill Assumption (A5).

Another comment on (A5)

I still have not given an explanation of the final assumption, (A5). But we are now ready for it, as we have some basic understanding of the Jacobian and the associated eigenvalues. What the assumption states is that the Jacobian evaluated at the DFE only has eigenvalues with *negative* real parts, i.e. the system is stable if $\mathscr{F}(x) = 0$. This means that not only the transmission side of the system is stable, but also the transmission-independent part of the system. We could, for example, imagine a model according to which there is constant, unchecked growth in one or more compartments. We could achieve that by allowing N_1 and N_2 to vary and having the mortality rates *larger* than the renewal rates. In that case, the system would not be stable, as its state would constantly change even in absence of infection. On page 174, I am referring to a possible relationship between (A5) and the statement that only systems are to be considered "that are stable in the absence of new infections." This is actually a very similar requirement to (A5), only a little less restrictive: While (A5) demands local (i.e. close to the DFE) stability of the whole system, the latter statement allows for systems that might be unstable if $\mathscr{F}(x) > 0$.

A short discourse on complex eigenvalues

Assumption (A5) is interesting for yet another reason: It mentions eigenvalues with *negative real parts*. This clearly indicates that there are eigenvalues with *imaginary* parts. I will not–and *could* not–embark on a comprehensive discourse on *complex eigenvalues*. I only will point out important aspects of complex eigenvalues that will dispel some of the mystique of that topic. I direct interested readers to many excellent resources, both off- and online (e.g. http://ocw.mit.edu/courses/mathematics/18-03sc-differential-equations-fall-2011/).

Complex eigenvalues arise when the characteristic equation has complex roots. Consider, for example, the characteristic equation

$$p(\lambda) = \lambda^2 - 2\lambda + 5. \tag{7.74}$$

Using the *quadratic formula*, we obtain the two solutions:

$$\frac{-2 \pm \sqrt{-16}}{2} = -1 \pm 2i. \tag{7.75}$$

To readers having difficulties understanding Eq. (7.75), I recommend a basic review of complex numbers.

If the eigenvalues are complex, we will still get a solution for a linear system of two differential equations $\dot{x} = Ax$, given an eigenvalue $\lambda = -1 + 2i$ such as

$$x = e^{(-1+2i)t}\mathbf{v} \tag{7.76}$$

where $\mathbf{v}$ is the corresponding eigenvector. That eigenvector will also be complex. Now we can take advantage of the following, extremely useful trigonometric identity

$$e^{it} = \cos t + i \sin t. \tag{7.77}$$

Applying this to (7.76), we get

$$\begin{aligned} e^{(-1+2i)t} &= e^{-t}e^{i2t} \\ &= e^{-t}(\cos 2t + i \sin t). \end{aligned} \tag{7.78}$$

This is instructive for two reasons:

1. The real part of the eigenvalue, -1, ends up in the factor e^{-t}. With increasing t the expression thus diminishes toward zero.
2. The imaginary part goes to the trigonometric expression, $\cos 2t + i \sin 2t$.

Now we can take advantage of another fact regarding complex solutions: If $x = \mathbf{x_1} + i\mathbf{x_2}$ is a solution to the system $\dot{x} = Ax$, then so are $\mathbf{x_1}$ and $\mathbf{x_2}$. The solution will be a product of a trigonometric expression (7.78) and the complex eigenvector. The complex solution will be treated as just outlined, resulting in two *real* solutions that contain trigonometric terms. The imaginary part of a complex eigenvalue therefore has something to do with a periodic behavior of the system.

7.3.2 Lemma 1—getting ready for R_0

Right after stating the five assumptions, van den Driessche and Watmough state the following lemma which will be needed for deriving an expression for R_0:

Lemma 1. If x_0 is a DFE of (7.30) and $f(x_0)$ satisfies (A1)–(A5), then the derivatives $D\mathscr{F}(x_0)$ and $D\mathscr{V}(x_0)$ are partitioned as

$$D\mathscr{F}(x_0) = \begin{pmatrix} F & 0 \\ 0 & 0 \end{pmatrix}, \qquad D\mathscr{V}(x_0) = \begin{pmatrix} V & 0 \\ J_3 & J_4 \end{pmatrix},$$

where F and V are the $m \times m$ matrices defined by

$$F = \left[\frac{\partial \mathscr{F}_i}{\partial x_j}(x_0)\right] \text{ and } V = \left[\frac{\partial \mathscr{V}_i}{\partial x_j}(x_0)\right] \text{ with } 1 \le i, j \le m.$$

Further, F is non-negative, V is a non-singular M-matrix and all eigenvalues of J_4 have positive real part.

So the partitioning of $D\mathcal{F}(x_0)$ and $D\mathcal{V}(x_0)$ is according to infected and not infected compartments.

Question 7.o

Write down $D\mathcal{F}(x_0)$ and $D\mathcal{V}(x_0)$ for our model.

The authors offer a relatively accessible proof of Lemma 1 which I will not discuss here. I will leave it at the following two comments.

1. An M-matrix is a square matrix with certain properties, the important one here is its *non-singularity*. A matrix that is non-singular can be inverted. This will be important for the derivation of R_0.
2. The reason for the fact that all eigenvalues of J_4 have *positive real part* can be understood from the following facts:
   - The eigenvalues of a block tridiagonal matrix such as
   $$Df(x_0) = D\mathcal{F}(x_0) - D\mathcal{V}(x_0) = \begin{pmatrix} F-V & 0 \\ -J_3 & -J_4 \end{pmatrix},$$
   are the eigenvalues of the diagonal blocks which are $F - V$ and $-J_4$. We therefore know that the eigenvalues of $-J_4$ also are eigenvalues of $Df(x_0)$.
   - As we know, by assumption, that all the eigenvalues of $Df(x_0)$ have *negative real* parts and the eigenvalues of a $-J_4$ also must by eigenvalues of $Df(x_0)$, they must only have *negative* real parts.
   - As the (real parts) of the eigenvalues $-J_4$ are *negative*, the eigenvalues of $-(-J_4) = J_4$ *must* only have *positive* real parts.

7.3.3 *Finally:* R_0

Finally, we are getting to the most important part of this paper, the one developing a general expression for the basic reproduction number R_0 based on the framework we just saw developed. Van den Driessche and Watmough use the nice notation $\mathcal{R}_0$ for that quantity, but we will stick to the more humble—although, admittedly, much less aesthetically pleasing—version R_0, simply to stay consistent. The authors embark on their discussion of the concept by the definition we already encountered on page 158 in the first article we discussed in this chapter [1]: R_0 is

> *"the expected number of secondary cases produced, in a completely susceptible population, by a typical infective individual."*

Van den Driessche and Watmough then point out the threshold quality of R_0 which we are already aware of:

> *"If $R_0 < 1$, then on average an infected individual produces less than one new infected individual over the course of its infectious period, and the infection cannot grow."*

> *"[I]f $R_0 > 1$, then each infected individual produces, on average, more than one new infection, and the disease can invade the population."*

They also remind us—although we have not seen this simple equality explicitly—that for the simplest compartmental models the basic reproduction number simply is the product of the infection rate with the duration of infection.

Question 7.p

How can we show that, in a simple compartmental SIR (= susceptible–infectious–removed) model, R_0 is the product of the infection rate with the duration of infection? Do you see an inaccuracy in this procedural definition of R_0?

For more complicated models we need a more general R_0 definition, though. Van den Driessche and Watmough propose:

Definition. A more general basic reproduction number can be defined as the number of new infections produced by a typical infective individual in a population at a DFE.

> *"To determine the fate of a –typically– infective individual introduced into the population, we consider the dynamics of the linearized system (7.46) with reinfection turned off." (p. 33)*

The term "reinfection turned off" is actually not very clear. What is meant is "transmission turned off". Considering model (7.30) with $\mathcal{F}(x)$ eliminated—which is the only model component representing transmission—and used in (7.46), we get

$$\dot{x} = -D\mathcal{V}(x_0)(x - x_0). \tag{7.79}$$

The negative sign results if $\mathcal{F}(x)$ is subtracted from (7.30); the negative sign does not go away when taking partial derivatives. As $\mathcal{V}$ captures the transfer between compartments (other than the *addition* due to infection), (7.79) should be helpful in characterizing the "fate" of an infectious individual introduced to DFE, in terms of time spent where.

Van den Driessche and Watmough then define $\psi_i(0)$ as the number of infected individuals initially in compartment i and $\psi(t) = (\psi_1(t), \ldots, \psi_m(t))^T$ is the number of initially infected remaining in each compartment at time t. Note that the vector $\psi(t)$ has length m as infected individuals can only "live" in the first m compartments.

As $\dot{x} = -D\mathcal{V}(x_0)(x - x_0)$ and, in our reduced model, $x_i = \psi_i$ for $i = 1, \ldots, m$, we can also write

$$\dot{\psi} = -\left.\begin{pmatrix} \partial\mathcal{V}_1/\partial x_1 & \ldots & \partial\mathcal{V}_1/\partial x_m \\ \vdots & \ddots & \vdots \\ \partial\mathcal{V}_m/\partial x_1 & \ldots & \partial\mathcal{V}_m/\partial x_m \end{pmatrix}\right|_{x_0} (\psi(t) - x_0^*) \tag{7.80}$$

$$= -V\psi(t). \tag{7.81}$$

The matrix in (7.80) is the left-upper $m \times m$ quadrant of $D\mathcal{V}$. This can be equated with V. Eq. (7.81) follows from (7.80) because the system is still close to the DFE and $x_0^* = 0$ for $x^* = (x_1, \ldots, x_m)^T$. The importance of (7.81) lies in the fact that we can directly solve it for ψ, again using the standard method for linear differential equations:

$$\psi(t) = e^{-Vt}\psi(0). \tag{7.82}$$

By knowing $\phi(t)$ we have characterized how the infectious move through the system. Now, at every point in time, if we put the transmission function, $\mathscr{F}$, back in place, we can figure out at what rate new infections are produced: We simply multiply, again just the upper $m \times m$ quadrant, of $D\mathscr{F}(x_0)$, which is F with the numbers still infected, ψ,

$$\dot{i} = F\psi(t) = Fe^{-Vt}\psi(0). \tag{7.83}$$

I use the symbol i to refer to the vector of the cumulative numbers of infected by the *index case(s)* in compartments $1, \ldots, m$. Clearly, to figure out the total number becoming infected we can integrate (7.83) with respect to time t, from 0 to infinity:

$$\begin{aligned}
\int_0^\infty i dt &= \int_0^{\int} Fe^{-Vt}\psi(0)dt \\
&= F\psi(0)\int_0^\infty e^{-Vt}dt \text{ (F and $\psi(0)$ are constants)} \\
&= F\psi(0)\left(-V^{-1}e^{-Vt}\right)\Big|_0^\infty \text{ (integrating exponential function)} \\
&= F\psi(0)\left(-0 + V^{-1}\right) \text{ (calculating definite integral)} \\
&= FV^{-1}\psi(0) \text{ (rearranging).}
\end{aligned} \tag{7.84}$$

Eq. (7.84) captures the number of infections produced by the index cases $\psi(0)$. V^{-1} is the inverse of V and because of this the fact that V is an M-matrix and thus invertible was important.

This is exactly equivalent to Diekmann et al.'s expression (7.10), $\mathbf{A_S}\ \mathbf{\Phi_0}$, only here we have been using FV^{-1} instead of $\mathbf{A_S}$ and $\psi(0)$ instead of $\mathbf{\Phi_0}$. We called $\mathbf{A_S}$ the *next-generation matrix* and, by analogy, FV^{-1} is the next-generation matrix, too. Had we started with *typical* index cases, (7.84) would represent R_0. Instead, however, we just started with *any* index case. But departing from FV^{-1} we can use the method of Diekmann et al. using the spectral radius of the next-generation matrix for R_0, i.e.

$$R_0 = \rho(FV^{-1}), \tag{7.85}$$

where ρ is the spectral radius of a square matrix, i.e. is the largest (real part) of the eigenvalues.

Question 7.q

Calculate the basic reproduction number R_0 for our model, (7.68)–(7.71).

This derivation of a general expression for R_0 is followed by the statement of

Theorem 2. Consider the disease transmission model given by (7.30) with $f(x)$ satisfying conditions (A1)–(A5). If x_0 is a DFE of the model, then x_0 is locally asymptotically stable if $R_0 < 1$, but unstable if $R_0 > 1$, where R_0 is defined by (7.85).

This is not really surprising, it is just a formal statement regarding the threshold quality of R_0 which is then rigorously proven, using matrix properties, especially of M-matrices. The interested reader may study that proof, but I will, instead, continue to the last two topics of this chapter, treating both of them relatively briefly.

7.3.4 Again: A vector–host model

On page 164 I commented on the discussion by Diekmann and colleagues on their treatment of vector-borne disease, under the ominous section title "A somewhat unfortunate choice of an example." I criticized their conceptualization of a basic reproduction number for a vector-borne system, arguing that vectors are not just another class of host, but, rather, an essential element in the chain of transmission. After presenting a series of example models, van den Driessche and Watmough also pick up the topic of vector-borne transmission and present the following model of a mosquito-borne disease, based on a published paper [2]:

$$\begin{aligned} \dot{I} &= \beta_s - (b+\gamma)I, &(7.86)\\ \dot{V} &= \beta_m MI - cV, &(7.87)\\ \dot{S} &= b - bs + \gamma I - \beta_s SV, &(7.88)\\ \dot{M} &= c - cM - \beta_m MI. &(7.89) \end{aligned}$$

The variables I and S represent infected and susceptible humans, respectively, and V and M are infected and uninfected mosquitoes. The parameters β_x and β_m are transmission parameters that not only capture the mosquito human-biting rate, but also the probability of human and mosquito infection, respectively; γ is reversion of humans to a susceptible state[5]; b and c are human and mosquito mortality rates. Treating this model as we discussed before, they formulate

$$F = \begin{pmatrix} o & \beta_s \\ \beta_m & 0 \end{pmatrix}, \qquad V = \begin{pmatrix} b+\gamma & 0 \\ 0 & c \end{pmatrix}. \qquad (7.90)$$

The choice of the label V for infected mosquitoes is unfortunate because of the duplication of the symbol for the matrix V—the choice of "good" symbols really can become challenging!

[5] In the case of *dengue*, after malaria the most important mosquito-borne disease, a person infected with a particular serotype—there are four—will be immune for life against that serotype. A person will, however, still be susceptible to the *other* serotypes, making him/her at risk for more severe forms of the disease upon "reinfection".

From this, they derive the formula for the basic reproduction number,

$$R_0 = \sqrt{\frac{\beta_s \beta_m}{c(b+\gamma)}}, \tag{7.91}$$

which exactly corresponds to the formulation by Diekmann et al. in Eq. (7.17), allowing for the different symbols. This agreement clearly appears to disqualify my criticism. The formulation of R_0 by van den Driessche and Watmough clearly qualifies it as a threshold parameter. For a threshold parameter that is 1 at the threshold, the square root does not matter ($\sqrt{1} = 1$). Yet, I still dispute whether it is—meaningfully—true to their definition of the basic reproduction number. Also, note that (7.91) is very similar to the square root of Macdonald's R_0 expression (see Chap. 5). I also refer the reader back to my discussion on page 165. So here, towards the very end of this book, it may be a good place for some—quite informal—deliberations that I find very important:

> Readers who almost made it through this book may have wondered about the many times when I pointed out inaccuracies, if not errors, in the papers we have discussed. At the time when I am writing these lines, the current paper, according to Google Scholar (https://scholar.google.com/scholar?q=van+den+driesche&btnG=&hl=en&as_sdt=0%2C11) has been cited over 2,300 times, which is a very impressive track record. As comparison, the key paper by Kermack and McKendrick [5] we discussed in Chap. 4 and which was written 65 years earlier, was cited just over 3,800 times. Pointing out "inaccuracies" in such a famed paper or being critical to some aspects certainly may be seen as heresy by some. What I believe is crucial, however, is to develop a critical attitude even towards papers that have almost scripture status. Intimidatingly obscure presentation should not be a deterrent to scrutiny by the interested reader. I certainly invite scrutiny of this book, too.

7.3.5 Final remarks

The paper by van den Driessche and Watmough references in its title "sub-threshold endemic equilibria". Such *sub-threshold endemic equilibria* would manifest in the stable existence of transmission in a given system despite $R_0 < 1$. Intuitively, this may appear possible, for example, when a model with many population subgroups allows for constant transmission in just *one* group, but is prohibitive to transmission in all the other, such that, on average, transmission is not sustained. This clearly is a very interesting problem. Van den Driessche and Watmough use tools of *center manifold theory* to address this problem in the context of their general model at DFE. Center manifold theory is a powerful, yet mathematically challenging, set of tools for the analysis of system stability and bifurcation phenomena. I do not claim to fully master these tools, but understand that existence of a center manifold requires a system that is not *hyperbolic*. Hyperbolicity of a system refers to the fact that all eigenvalues of the Jacobian have *non-zero* real parts. Assumption (A5) specifically requires all eigenvalues of the Jacobian to have negative real parts (see p. 172). This would appear to preclude the existence of a center manifold and thus the application of center manifold theory methods. I will leave the continuation of this analysis to the future.

Appendix 7.A Answers

7.a This is, once again, not a completely straightforward question, as there may not be one universally accepted best answer. The two issues I was thinking of are:

- Remember that in ODE models of the Kermack & McKendrick type there are no individuals! We are dealing with a continuous quantity. Even though very large population could, conceivably, be well approximated with the "gas analogy", talking about individuals, as I did, is technically inappropriate.
- In this context, there is no probability: These are, after all, deterministic models.

In all fairness, however, especially with regard to the first issue ("individual"), regardless of the nature of the model, the process that is modeled does involve individuals!

7.b The h-state variable is not only denoted by ξ, but it is also in the term $A(\tau, \xi, \eta)$ assigned the value ξ. What I referred to as inconsistency is the use of the same symbol for a variable as well as for a specific value for that variable. That can lead to confusion!
The second "inconsistency" (maybe better, lack of precision) is the term "expected infectivity": the adjective "expected" is a heavily charged term in statistics, as in *expected value* (mean). The use of this word in the context of deterministic models is, in my opinion, misguided.

7.c The next-generation factor is given by the expression

$$\sum_{\eta\in\Omega} S(\xi) \int_0^\infty A(\tau, \xi, \eta)\, d\tau.$$

Before deriving that quantity I posed the question: "How many people will an infectious individual of h-type η produce in total?"—The next-generation factor represents exactly that number:

1. For each h-type ξ being a recipient of the infection, the total amount of infectivity received–over the whole infectious period of the "infection donor"–is calculated using the definite integral of $A(\tau, \xi, \eta)$ with respect to time. For most infections, if not all, the infectious period may be days, sometimes even weeks or years. The upper limit of infinity (∞) therefore may appear unnecessary. The reason for that choice is the intent to include all possible infectious times; this way we can be absolutely sure. The resulting quantity, $\int_0^\infty A(\tau, \xi, \eta)\, d\tau$ thus represents the full "amount" of infectivity caused in one susceptible individual of type ξ (can be anything in Ω, the universe of h-types) by our infectious individual of h-type η.
2. If $\int_0^\infty A(\tau, \xi, \eta)\, d\tau$ is multiplied by $S(\xi)$, which is the number of susceptibles of h-type ξ, we obtain the total "number" of infections (the quotes are used for the

same reason I sometimes use quotes in this context; see, e.g., answer to Question 7.a) caused in all $S(\xi)$ individuals of h-type ξ.

3. If this procedure is repeated for all values of ξ and the resulting quantities are added, we therefore arrive at the total amount of infectivity (aka numbers of infections) caused by one infectious individual of h-type η in the whole population.

7.d The ηth column of $\mathbf{A_S}$ is

$$\mathbf{A}_\eta = \begin{bmatrix} a_{1\eta}\, S(1) \\ a_{2\eta}\, S(2) \\ \vdots \\ a_{n\eta}\, S(n) \end{bmatrix}. \tag{7.92}$$

All elements of this vector are positive because a_{ij} denote the number of infections generated, and $S(k)$ mean the number of susceptible individuals of h-type k–thus they equal their absolute value. Thus, the L_1-norm is just the sum of these values:

$$\sum_{\xi=1}^{n} S(\xi)\, a_{\xi\eta},$$

which is the next-generation factor (7.3).

7.e The fundamental "problem" (the quotes will be explained below) with expression (7.11) lies in the fact that $\mathbf{A_S}$ is constant. Revisiting the definition of $\mathbf{A_S}$ as given in (7.8), we see that it is based on specific values of $S(\xi)$ which are the number of susceptibles of specific h-type (e.g. ξ). In any infectious disease outbreak, though, the number of susceptible individuals will decrease over time and thus from generation of infection to generation. If we remind ourselves that our purpose is to find the basic reproduction number R_0, we realize that this is not a "problem", but a direct implication of the definition of that quantity as:

> *"[...] the* expected number of secondary cases *produced, in a* completely susceptible population *[...]" (p. 365)*

The highlighted text points to the fact R_0 is, in a sense, a *theoretical* quantity, as no secondary cases can be produced without *reducing* the number of susceptibles. This is what Diekmann et al. mean when they write in the introduction section (p. 365):

> *"[...] we first of all* linearize, *i.e. we ignore the fact that the density of susceptibles decreases due to the infection process."*

7.f As $\mathbf{A_S}$ is a square matrix which is multiplied with itself n times, $\mathbf{A_S}^n$, it still is a square matrix of same dimensions. If a square matrix such as $\mathbf{A_S}^n$ is multiplied by a column vector, e.g. $\mathbf{\Phi}_0$, which has n elements, a column vector of same size results. Eq. (7.13) states that, in the "long run", regardless of the starting value of the vector, $\mathbf{\Phi}_0$ repeated multiplication with $\mathbf{A_S}$ converges to a specific vector, $\mathbf{\Phi}_d$, multiplied by a constant, c, and another quantity, ϱ_d, raised to the kth power–remember that we let k go to infinity. That is an interpretation of (7.13), although a quite "bloodless" one.

As for the second part of the question, relating to the fitting mathematical context: First, an important thing to note here is the fact that, once k becomes "large",

$$\mathbf{A_S}\boldsymbol{\Phi}_\mathbf{k} \approx \varrho_d \, \boldsymbol{\Phi}_\mathbf{k}. \tag{7.93}$$

This means that, for large k, multiplying $\mathbf{A_S}$ with $\boldsymbol{\Phi}_\mathbf{k}$ is basically equivalent to multiplying that vector with the number ϱ_d, which corresponds to the stretching or lengthening the vector. Furthermore,

$$\mathbf{A_S}\boldsymbol{\Phi}_\mathbf{d} = \varrho_d \, \boldsymbol{\Phi}_\mathbf{d}. \tag{7.94}$$

This clearly means that $\boldsymbol{\Phi}_\mathbf{d}$ is an eigenvector of $\mathbf{A_S}$ and ϱ_d the associated eigenvalue. In fact, ϱ_d is the *dominant* (thus the subscript d) or largest eigenvalue of that matrix. This is nicely derived in [7] (see online supplement for demonstration). Moreover, the eigenvalue *must* be a *real* one because the eigenvector must also consist of *real and non-negative* numbers (numbers of individuals). If you are not familiar with eigenvalues and eigenvectors, or even with linear algebra in general, there are countless resources on- and offline that give sufficient basic introductions into the topic. At least superficial familiarity with linear algebra is important to following this chapter.

7.g If the outer integral with respect to η, i.e. the h-type of the *infecting* individual, is replaced by a sum, we obtain

$$S(\xi)\sum_{\eta\in\Omega}\int_0^\infty A(\tau,\xi,\eta)d\tau\phi(\eta) = S(\xi)\sum_{\eta\in\Omega} a_{\xi\eta}\phi(\eta). \tag{7.95}$$

Recall that the ξth row of the next generation matrix (7.8) is

$$(a_{\xi,1}S(\xi), a_{\xi,2}S(\xi), \ldots, a_{\xi,n}S(\xi)).$$

This is a row vector, and the sum over that vector (its L_1-norm) is

$$\sum_{\eta=1}^{n} a_{\xi,\eta}S(\xi);$$

this is quantity we were looking for (7.3).

7.h The spectral radius $r(K(S))$ represents the per-generation growth factor of the epidemic (under linearization) as we have seen in Sect. 7.2.1 and in expression (7.18). Therefore, if that factor is below 1, the epidemic will vanish; if it is larger than 1, it will explode. The "lengthening" and "shortening" property of $r(K(S))$ at least suggests that the spectral radius may represent an eigenvalue.

7.i There are differences in the two expressions that are directly tied to the different assumptions: The inner integral of (7.21), $\int_0^\infty A(\tau,\xi,\eta)i(t-\tau,\eta)d\tau$, is replaced by the sum $a_{\xi,1}I(t,1) + a_{\xi,2}I(t,2) + \cdots + a_{\xi,n}I(t,n)$. We can do this as, according to our assumption regarding the constant infectiousness, only the number of infectious individuals, not their history, matters. Eq. (7.22) is, in fact, a *linear* first-order differential equation. As we have seen before, transmission processes are fundamentally *nonlinear*. Why we are, nevertheless, faced with a linear equation here is the *linearization* of the system I referred to in the last sentence before the question. This is what

I referred to as "funny": The forcing of the number of susceptibles, here by h-type, to be *constant*. Linearization, however, is a valid and often used technique to simplify complex systems.

7.j The most important characteristics for a transmission model are defined with respect to the transmission process, such as "susceptible", "infectious" and "removed". This simple setup would cover the "Kermack & McKendrick model" which we are familiar with. We could expand this simple model, for example, to accommodate different levels of susceptibility or infectiousness. We could also introduce different stages of the disease that might be associated with different levels of infectiousness or mortality, etc. The sky is the limit to the modeler's creativity!

7.k Considering the transmission model described by three (or four!) different sets of equations ((7.32)–(7.35), (7.36)–(7.39), and (7.41)–(7.43); (7.44)), Eqs. (7.36)–(7.39) are best suited to our attempt to extract the two (vectors of) functions, $\mathscr{F}$ and $\mathscr{V}$. As each of the two functions is defined for any compartment, they can be indexed, in our case, by 1 through 4. Consulting the definition of $\mathscr{F}$ (appearance of new infections), we first realize that for the *uninfected* compartments, i.e. compartments 3 and 4 (Eqs. (7.38) and (7.39)), the functions $\mathscr{F}_3$ and $\mathscr{F}_4$ are zero, i.e.

$$\begin{aligned}\mathscr{F}_3 &= 0,\\ \mathscr{F}_4 &= 0.\end{aligned}$$

We already knew this, of course (Assumption (A3)); I also already stated it after the third version of the model. $\mathscr{F}_1$ and $\mathscr{F}_2$ are a little more interesting, though. New infectious are generated by the positive terms of Eqs. (7.36) and (7.37), $\beta_{11}x_1x_3 + \beta_{21}x_2x_3$ and $\beta_{12}x_1x_4 + \beta_{22}x_2x_4$. The only way of adding to compartments 1 and 2 is to turn residents of compartments 3 and 4, respectively, to *new* infections. It does not have to be that way; a model could be formulated according to which, for example, a change between infectious compartments were admissible.
As for $\mathscr{V} = \mathscr{V}^- - \mathscr{V}^+$, which corresponds to the net change in compartments, by processes other than *adding* new infections (the business of function $\mathscr{F}$), we realize that in our simple model there are only two other ways to move *out of compartments*:

1. Moving out of compartments 1 and 2, due to *removal*, i.e. losing infectiousness (Eqs. (7.36) and (7.37), $\mathscr{V}_1^- = x_1\mu_1$ and $\mathscr{V}_2^- = x_2\mu_2$). By the way, what happens to those "people"? We simply omitted the "removal compartments" as they are redundant (see p. 172).
2. Moving out of compartments 3 and 4 because of infection–thus the corresponding functions are $\mathscr{V}_3^- = \beta_{11}x_1x_3 + \beta_{21}x_2x_3$ and $\mathscr{V}_4^- = \beta_{12}x_1x_4 + \beta_{22}x_2x_4$.

Because our model does not allow for the movement between compartments, except for newly infected being "transferred" to compartments 1 or 2, and there is no birth or immigration, all the $\mathscr{V}^+$s are equal to zero. All this implies that

$$\begin{aligned}\mathscr{V}_1 &= \mathscr{V}_1^-,\\ \mathscr{V}_2 &= \mathscr{V}_2^-,\end{aligned}$$

$$\begin{aligned}\mathcal{V}_3 &= \mathcal{V}_3^-,\\ \mathcal{V}_4 &= \mathcal{V}_4^-.\end{aligned}$$

7.1 Applying Eq. (7.45) to $f(x) = x^2$, we get

$$l(x) = a^2 + 2a\,(a - x),$$

where $a = 3$ ("in the neighborhood of 3"). Note that we have switched the '$\approx$' sign for the "=" sign, but replaced $f(x)$ by $l(x)$ for "linear approximation". So plugging-in the three values, we get:

$$\begin{aligned}l(3.1) &= 3^2 + 2 \times 3\,(3.1 - 3) = 9.6,\\ l(3.2) &= 9 + 6 \times 0.2 = 10.2,\\ l(4) &= 9 + 6 \times 1 = 15.\end{aligned}$$

By comparing these "estimates" with the *true* values, we have

Function	Estimate	True value
3.1^2	9.6	9.61
3.2^2	10.2	10.24
4^2	15	16

Clearly, for values close to 3, the approximated value is quite good, but as we move away from 3 for the input, the approximation is getting progressively worse.

7.m Obviously, if we had $\dot{x}^*$ on the left-hand side of (7.53), we would have the exact equivalent of (7.50) with $x = x^*$ and $A = Df(x_0)$. We need to have the system in that form in order to use the formula for the general solution (7.51). If we write out $\dot{x}^*$ and use basic properties of derivatives, we get

$$\begin{aligned}\dot{x}^* &= \frac{d(x - x_0)}{dt}\\ &= \frac{dx}{dt} - \frac{dx_0}{dt}\\ &= \frac{dx}{dt} \text{ (the derivative of a constant, such as } \frac{dx_0}{dt}\text{, is zero)}\\ &= \dot{x}.\end{aligned}$$

We have thus established that $\dot{x} = \dot{x}^*$. We can therefore write (7.53) as

$$\dot{x}^* = Df(x_0)x^* \tag{7.96}$$

and use the result (7.51) we found for (7.50) also for (7.46).

7.n The "problem" with the first model (7.36)–(7.39) was, loosely speaking, the fact that absolutely nothing was going on in compartments x_3 and x_4, and actually in the whole system, as long as the infected compartments stayed empty. Even if we added a few—or even very many—to x_3 or x_4, the system would remain completely static. This situation, where some eigenvalues have *zero* real parts, is covered by *center manifold theory* which is a powerful, but difficult mathematical method which is also used by van den Driessche and Watmough in the second part of their paper. We will only briefly touch on that.

7.o The Jacobian $Df(x_0)$ is the matrix of partial derivatives for the whole model and is the sum of $D\mathcal{F}(x_0)$ and $-D\mathcal{V}(x_0)$ or, less obscurely stated,

$$Df(x_0) = D\mathcal{F}(x_0) - D\mathcal{V}(x_0). \tag{7.97}$$

This is merely due to the fact that

$$f_i(x) = \mathcal{F}_i(x) - \mathcal{V}_i(x).$$

If we take partial derivatives on both sides of the equation with respect to all variables $(x_1, \ldots, x_4)$ and do this for all functions $(f_1, \ldots, f_4)$ we obtain (7.97). On the other hand, if we start with the Jacobian (7.72),

$$Df(x_0) = \begin{bmatrix} \beta_{11}x_3 - (\gamma_1 + \mu_1) & \beta_{21}x_3 & 0 & 0 \\ \beta_{12}x_4 & \beta_{22}x_4 - (\gamma_2 - \mu_2) & 0 & 0 \\ -\beta_{11}x_3 - \rho_1 & -\beta_{21}x_3 & -\mu_1 & 0 \\ -\beta_{12}x_4 & -\beta_{22}x_4 - \rho_2 & 0 & -\mu_2 \end{bmatrix},$$

we should be able to extract $D\mathcal{F}(x_0)$ and $D\mathcal{V}(x_0)$ by considering where the different expressions were derived from. So starting out with $D\mathcal{F}(x_0)$ we already know, from Lemma 1, that its upper left 2×2 partition is F, which is the only non-zero partition of that matrix. The expressions of F must derive from the transmission process that adds to the infected compartments, x_1 and x_2. Those must be *positive* expressions because infection is the only way anything is added to these compartments.[6] These expressions are easy to spot, and we can construct

$$F = \begin{pmatrix} \beta_{11}x_3 & \beta_{21} \\ \beta_{12}x_4 & \beta_{22}x_4 \end{pmatrix}. \tag{7.98}$$

This immediately leads to V, as this must be everything we left out from the left upper corner of $Df(x_0)$ to obtain F,

$$V = \begin{pmatrix} \gamma_1 + \mu_1 & 0 \\ 0 & \gamma_2 - \mu_2 \end{pmatrix}. \tag{7.99}$$

The two other partitions of $D\mathcal{V}(x_0)$ can be directly taken from the lower left 2×2 and the lower right 2×2 partitions of the Jacobian as there is no contribution of $D\mathcal{F}(x_0)$ (there are only zeros there). Let me therefore just write down J_4,

$$J_4 = \begin{pmatrix} -\mu_1 & 0 \\ 0 & -\mu_2 \end{pmatrix}. \tag{7.100}$$

7.p To answer this question, we first write down a really simple model:

$$\dot{x} = -\beta x y, \tag{7.101}$$
$$\dot{y} = \beta x y - \gamma y, \tag{7.102}$$
$$\dot{z} = \gamma y. \tag{7.103}$$

[6] That does not have to be true, of course, but holds for our model.

Similar to the notation for the model (7.32)–(7.35), etc., x represents the susceptibles and y the infectious class, β is the transmission coefficient and γ is the removal parameter. Furthermore, we explicitly keep track of the *removed* class, z.
As we have seen, R_0 is a threshold parameter, and if $R_0 = 1$, i.e. when we are exactly at the threshold, the epidemic will neither grow, nor die down,[7] i.e. "nothing changes". In terms of a differential equation model, this means that the left-hand side derivatives, $\dot{x}$, $\dot{y}$, and $\dot{z}$, can be set to zero:

$$0 = -\beta N, \tag{7.104}$$

$$0 = \beta N - \gamma, \tag{7.105}$$

$$0 = \gamma. \tag{7.106}$$

Note that I have replaced xy with N because, by definition, we are dealing with a *fully susceptible* population, thus $x = N$; furthermore, we are considering *one* infectious individual. As all three Eqs. (7.104)–(7.106) equal 0, we can equate them, specifically let me equate (7.104) and (7.106):

$$\beta N = \gamma. \tag{7.107}$$

Dividing both sides by γ, we obtain

$$\frac{\beta N}{\gamma} = 1. \tag{7.108}$$

The left-hand side of (7.108) evaluates to 1 at the threshold we are interested in, so we can call this quantity R_0, i.e.

$$R_0 = \frac{\beta N}{\gamma}.$$

The numerator represents the *infection rate*, while $\frac{1}{\gamma} = \gamma^{-1}$ is the *mean duration of infection*.
The inaccuracy I was referring to can be found in van den Driessche and Watmough's description of the numerator as *the* infection rate; it should be described as the rate of infection if the population is fully susceptible, i.e. $x = N$, and if there is just one infectious, i.e. $y = 1$. Also, the *mean duration of infection* brings up, once again, the mixing of a statistical term into the deterministic framework.

7.q To begin we only need the two 2×2 matrices, F and V. Fortunately, we have already written down those two matrices in answering Question 7.o: For F, see (7.98),

$$F = \begin{pmatrix} \beta_{11}x_3 & \beta_{21} \\ \beta_{12}x_4 & \beta_{22}x_4 \end{pmatrix},$$

and for V, by (7.99),

$$V = \begin{pmatrix} \gamma_1 + \mu_1 & 0 \\ 0 & \gamma_2 - \mu_2 \end{pmatrix}.$$

[7] In the context of this "closed model" where there is no influx of new susceptibles, any outbreak *has* to eventually die down. But it may hold for the linearized case (no depletion of susceptibles).

Now we have to invert V. As we are only dealing with a 2×2 matrix, we can use the formula for inverting a matrix $A = \begin{pmatrix} a & b \\ c & d \end{pmatrix}$:

$$A^{-1} = \frac{1}{|A|}\begin{pmatrix} d & -b \\ -c & a \end{pmatrix} = \frac{1}{ad - bc}\begin{pmatrix} d & -b \\ -c & a \end{pmatrix}, \tag{7.109}$$

where $|A|$ is the determinant of A. Applying this formula to our matrix V, we get

$$V^{-1} = \frac{1}{(\gamma_1 + \mu_1)(\gamma_2 - \mu_2)}\begin{pmatrix} \gamma_2 - \mu_2 & 0 \\ 0 & \gamma_1 + \mu_1 \end{pmatrix} = \begin{pmatrix} \frac{1}{\gamma_1+\mu_1} & 0 \\ 0 & \frac{1}{\gamma_2-\mu_2} \end{pmatrix}. \tag{7.110}$$

Using this we can calculate

$$\begin{aligned} FV^{-1} &= \begin{pmatrix} \beta_{11}x_3 & \beta_{21} \\ \beta_{12}x_4 & \beta_{22}x_4 \end{pmatrix}\begin{pmatrix} \frac{1}{\gamma_1+\mu_1} & 0 \\ 0 & \frac{1}{\gamma_2-\mu_2} \end{pmatrix} \\ &= \begin{pmatrix} \frac{\beta_{11}x_3}{\gamma_1+\mu_1} & \frac{\beta_{21}}{\gamma_2-\mu_2} \\ \frac{\beta_{12}x_4}{\gamma_1+\mu_1} & \frac{\beta_{22}x_2}{\gamma_2-\mu_2} \end{pmatrix}. \end{aligned} \tag{7.111}$$

The final step is to calculate the eigenvalues and pick the largest one. Let me plug-in the values we have used before: Again using a computer to calculate the eigenvalues (see online Supplement) we get the two eigenvalues, 0.210 and 0.190. Therefore, $R_0 = 0.210$. This system clearly does not support epidemic transmission!

Appendix 7.B Supplementary material

Supplementary material related to this chapter can be found online at http://dx.doi.org/10.1016/B978-0-12-802260-3.00007-9.

References

[1] O. Diekmann, J. Heesterbeek, J.A. Metz, On the definition and the computation of the basic reproduction ratio R_0 in models for infectious diseases in heterogeneous populations, Journal of Mathematical Biology 28 (4) (1990) 365–382.
[2] Z. Feng, J.X. Velasco-Hernández, Competitive exclusion in a vector–host model for the dengue fever, Journal of Mathematical Biology 35 (5) (1997) 523–544.
[3] H.J.A.M. Heijmans, The dynamical behaviour of the age–size-distribution of a cell population, in: The Dynamics of Physiologically Structured Populations, in: Lecture Notes in Biomathematics, vol. 68, Springer, 1986, pp. 185–202, Chap. V.
[4] H.W. Hethcote, J.W. Van Ark, Epidemiological models for heterogeneous populations: proportionate mixing, parameter estimation, and immunization programs, Mathematical Biosciences 84 (1) (1987) 85–118.
[5] M. Kermack, A. McKendrick, Contributions to the mathematical theory of epidemics. Part I, Proceedings of the Royal Society A 115 (1927) 700–721.

[6] P. Van den Driessche, J. Watmough, Reproduction numbers and sub-threshold endemic equilibria for compartmental models of disease transmission, Mathematical Biosciences 180 (1) (2002) 29–48.

[7] E.W. Weisstein, Eigenvector, URL http://mathworld.wolfram.com/Eigenvector.html, 2002.

Index

Printed in the United States
By Bookmasters